What Rural Health Leaders Are Saying

Bill Auxier, Ph.D.

Monica,
Thank you
for your leadership!
- Bill A

What Rural Health Leaders Are Saying

Edited by: Morissa Schwartz

Cover Design Concept by: C5 Designs

ISBN: 978-0991631308

Table of Contents

Dedicated to

all the rural health leaders

who work long hours

and

wear many hats

serving the people

living in rural areas.

Special Thank You

to

R.D. Williams

for providing the inspiration

for the creation of the

Rural Health Leadership Radio™

podcast.

Thank you
to all the exceptional rural health thought leaders who have contributed to this book and made Rural Health Leadership Radio™ a reality.
(listed in alphabetical order)

Dr. Janelle Ali-Dinar
Kris Allen
Marc Augsburger
Dr. Steve Barnett
Teryl Eisinger
Terry Hill
Mike Huff
Dr. Mike Keegan
Ryan Kelly
Lisa Kilawee
Gary Lucas
Liz Monk
Alan Morgan
Cody Mullen
Brock Slabach
Dr. David Swenson
R.D. Williams

Introduction

Rural Health Leadership Radio™ is a weekly podcast hosted by me, Dr. Bill Auxier, that premiered August 2, 2016. Each week I interview rural health leaders from around the country as they discuss the important issues affecting the rural health community. My guests discuss everything from hospital closures and their effects on the community, to billing and coding, what it means to be a leader, and what rural health leaders could be doing better. Within these pages are most of the podcast interviews from the first five months, starting with the inaugural episode where I introduce myself and the goals of *Rural Health Leadership Radio™*.

The following pages contain some memorable moments, interviews, and lessons from the show.

You can check out the *Rural Health Leadership Radio™* podcast at www.rhlradio.com.

I'm Dr. Bill Auxier, and I welcome you to *What Rural Health Leaders Are Saying.*

What Rural Health Leaders Are Saying features leaders working in rural health, leaders of hospitals, leaders of clinics, of networks, of companies, communities, organizations. People in a lot of roles, but in leadership roles in rural health. All of them have been guests on the podcast, *Rural Health Leadership Radio™.*

Over the last ten years, nearly one hundred rural hospitals have closed their doors. When a rural hospital closes, it really has two major impacts in the community. The most obvious one, of course, is health care. If there's not a rural hospital close by and you have to drive to a larger city that's further away, there's risk to that, healthcare risk. Secondly, usually in a small town or smaller rural community, the hospital is one of the largest if not the largest employer in town. There's also an economic aspect of this and job loss aspect when a rural hospital closes its door. Now, roughly 1 in 3 rural hospitals has been identified as at risk.

If there's ever been a need for strong leadership, that time is now. That is part of *Rural Health Leadership Radio's*™ mission, to provide a forum to have conversations with rural health leaders to discuss and share ideas about what's working, what isn't working, and things that people have tried that haven't worked out the way they'd planned, therefore, a lesson learned. We want to talk about success stories and strategies and things to avoid and anything else that you want to hear about.

The idea behind the *Rural Health Leadership Radio™* podcast is to provide a forum that's absolutely free to anybody who wants to tune in and listen. The idea behind this book, *What Rural Health Leaders are Saying*, is to provide a different means of sharing these conversations. We're here to provide a voice for rural health and the primary investment is in your time. My goal is to make sure that you receive a huge return on your investment.

One question I ask every guest is, what is your definition of leadership? After all, *What Rural Health Leaders are Saying* is all about leadership.

My favorite definition of leadership is, leadership is what happens when others follow when they don't have to. I have to admit that's not my original definition of leadership, I stole it from Jim Collins. Jim Collins is a well know author who has written several books. *Good to Great* is the first book I ever read of his, an awesome book. He has also written *Built to Last* and *Great by Choice*. He is a prolific author and speaker. When you think about it, getting others to follow when they don't have to is a major statement of the type of leadership philosophy that one espouses. It is the opposite of an autocratic style of leadership where you give everyone orders. That's my favorite definition of leadership.

Why was *Rural Health Leadership Radio™* created? It was created to provide a forum. It all stems from a conversation I had with the CEO of a rural hospital in Florida. During a conversation with the CEO of a critical access hospital, I asked him, "What's one of the biggest challenges that you face as a rural health leader?" He said, "I really don't know what's going on in other hospitals. I don't know what other hospitals CEOs are doing. It's like we all guard our information closely, like it's a secret. I don't know what a CEO down the road is doing that's working and what's not working." He said, "I can find out what they're doing, but I have to spend time and money to find out by traveling and going to meetings or subscribing to services, that sort of thing. I don't always have time or money to receive that information."

I really thought about that. The following day, I was listening to a podcast when a light bulb went off. Why not start a podcast that allows rural health leaders, rural hospital CEOs, and other rural health leaders share information about what's working and what's not working. Talk about low cost and easy, that's the reason *Rural Health Leadership Radio™* was started. To accomplish that goal. To share information, to share best practices and to help rural health leaders become more effective.

My career in healthcare started when I was in high school and I have been working in healthcare ever since. In high school, everyone, especially my junior and senior year, were asking, "What are you going to do when you graduate?" I had an inkling that I wanted to go into healthcare, but the only thing I knew about healthcare was what I had experienced as a kid, as a patient, when I was hurt or sick or injured. I was curious about healthcare as an occupation. I always like to joke and say, "I got so sick and tired of people asking me what I was going to do after I graduated from high school that I ended up in our local hospital." The only thing was, I was in the local hospital applying for a job.

The pragmatic side of me said, "Hey, if you want to learn about healthcare, why don't you try to get a job at the hospital and learn about healthcare." That's what I did. My first job in healthcare was that of a nurse's aide in the small hospital in our community. The community I grew up in, the entire county, had around 10,000 people and that's true to this day. It's a very rural area in southern Illinois. McLeansboro is the town and we had a small hospital, Hamilton Memorial Hospital. That's where I received my first job in healthcare as a nurse's aide.

I went on to college, and I ended up majoring in business. Upon graduation, I worked on the industry side of healthcare. I worked for medical device companies and surgical device companies, working my way up in each organization until I became the CEO of surgical device manufacturer with worldwide distribution. I've had the opportunity to travel the world working in healthcare, exposed to a lot of different cultures, a lot of different issues, all focused on healthcare. At the same time, I continued my education; I received my bachelor's degree in business from the University of Evansville in Evansville, Indiana. Go Purple Aces! I received my master's degree in communication from Eastern Michigan University. Then I went on to receive my doctorate in leadership from Andrews University in Berrien Springs, Michigan.

I have real-world experience in leadership and academic training in leadership. Combining the two allows me to serve rural health leaders. Rural health is in my roots.

As a kid growing up, we needed that rural hospital, especially the way I tortured my little brother, Tony. I'll never forget, it's one of my first memories that I have as a kid. We were both little, I'm guessing I was 5 or 6 years old. The car was parked in front of the house and the windows were rolled down. I could crawl up into the car through the open window, but my little brother was too small to make that happen, but he wanted to crawl through the open window too. After I crawled up into the car, I told my brother, "Give me your arm." I yanked and pulled on his arm, trying to pull him up into the car until he started wailing and crying, so much so that mom came out to see what was happening. She rushed him to the hospital.

I had pulled his shoulder out of place. I wasn't trying to be malicious or anything. Mom was able to get him to the local hospital where they fixed him up, good as new. They relocated his shoulder, gave him some pain medication and shortly thereafter, he was feeling okay again.

Then there was the time when he was stung by a bee. None of us knew he was allergic to bee stings! Thank God, we had a hospital nearby, because it probably saved his life.

My dad was forced into early retirement. He was bi-vocational; a country preacher and he drove a truck for Standard Oil, selling and delivering their petroleum products to farmers. The Standard Oil job was the one that fed our family. Standard Oil made some major policy changes on how they did business in rural America, and delayed their decision for dad as long as they could, but finally forced him into early retirement. In his retirement, he took on all kinds of odd jobs at an age earlier than he had planned on, retiring at the age of fifty-six.

One of the things he got into was cutting firewood with his chainsaw. Oftentimes he would have back pain after working strenuously cutting wood. When that happened, he would come home and press his back against the door frame to relieve his back pain, until one day, that wasn't working anymore. Mom ran him out to Hamilton Memorial Hospital to the emergency room. What he didn't realize was that his back pain was due to the fact that he was having a heart attack! And he was having a heart attack right then! The ER staff stabilized him and transferred him to a larger nearby hospital in a larger town. If not for that rural hospital, God only knows what would have happened to him. It served a major purpose to keep him alive. If he would have had to travel to the big city hospital instead, the travel time would have made a huge difference.

Then there is my mother. Mom was diagnosed with ovarian cancer late in life. She had a tough time in her final days. She was a patient at Hamilton Memorial Hospital longer than any of us had planned. She was bedridden during her final stage in life. She had always been a huge gardener, not as a hobby, more out of necessity. Gardening was an economical way to feed our family. Gardening had become a way of life, so she continued gardening after all of us left home. While she was bedridden, I was so touched by this, some of the members of the church she belonged to came and planted a flower garden outside the window of her hospital room to give her some pleasure in her final days of life. In her final days she was able to see some of the glorious flowers and plants that God has given us on earth. I don't think you could've done that at a large urban hospital.

Rural hospitals play a definite role in healthcare. In Hamilton County, where I grew up, the hospital is the second largest employer in the county after the school system. If that hospital closed, not only would it be a devastating impact to the healthcare of everyone that resides there, it would be a devastating impact economically with the jobs it provides.

Many of the men and women who serve in the military are from rural settings. In my own family, my grandpa was in World War I, my dad was in World War II, and my brother was in Vietnam. Many veterans come from rural America. Keeping our rural hospitals open serves a major role in taking care of our veterans.

The goal of *What Rural Health Leaders Are Saying* is to share the dialogue from *Rural Health Leadership Radio™*. As you will see, I have had the privilege of interviewing some very interesting rural health leaders. In the pages that follow, you will read about their insights, their knowledge, their expertise on what's working, what's not working, lessons learned, their opinions, and what the future holds.

Alan Morgan

I was honored to have a conversation with the National Rural Health Association CEO, Alan Morgan. We delved into the risk of rural hospital closures and the dramatic forthcoming changes in rural health care. These topics are discussed separately and with regard to improving the health of rural communities, recruitment of health care providers and leaders, and collaborations within the NRHA to make projects and goals more successful in the future.

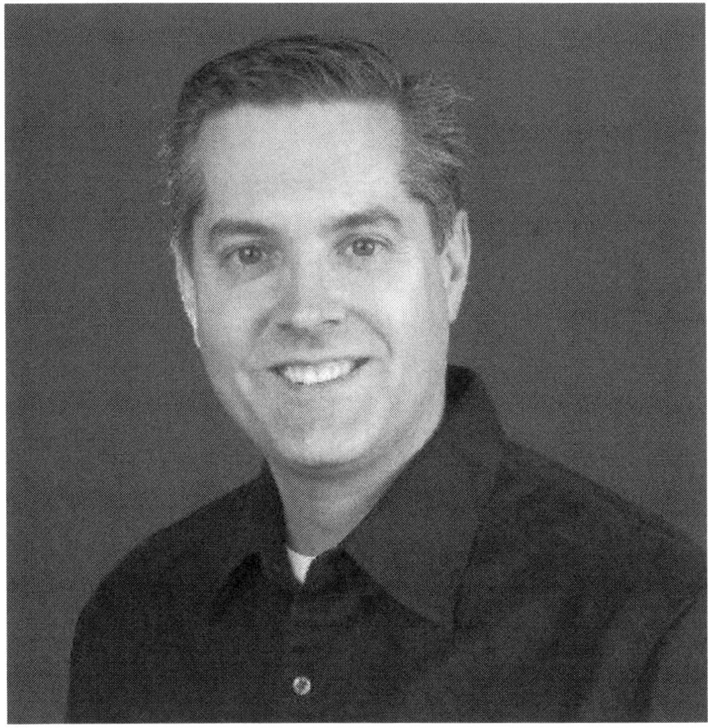

Bill: Alan Morgan, CEO of the National Rural Health Association (NRHA), is recognized as being among the top one hundred most influential people in health care by Modern Health Care magazine. He's been with the NRHA since 2001, and has served as it's CEO for the past eleven and a half years. He has more than twenty-six years of experience in health policy development at the state and federal level, and is one of the nation's leading experts on rural health policy.

Alan has served as a co-author for the publication, *Policy and Politics in Nursing and Healthcare*, and for the publication, *Rural Populations and Health*. In addition, his health policy articles have been published in numerous journals, including *The American Journal of Clinical Medicine, The Journal of Rural Health, The Journal of Cardiovascular Management, The Journal of Pacing and Clinical Electrophysiology, Cardiac Electrophysiology Review,* and in *Laboratory Medicine*.

Alan served as staff for the former U.S. congressman, Dick Nichols, and also for the former governor of Kansas, Mike Hayden. Additionally, his past experience includes ten years as a health care lobbyist for the American Society of Clinical Pathologists, The Heart Rhythm Society, and for VHA. He holds a bachelor's degree in journalism from the University of Kansas, and a master's degree in public administration from George Mason University. Welcome Alan!

Alan: Well, thank you very much, Bill. I appreciate the opportunity to join you.

Bill: I'm honored to have this conversation with you. The first question I have for you Alan is, how do you define leadership?

Alan: That definition is really going to vary from person to person. For me personally it's about the ability to define common goals, and then to enable your team to reach those goals together. By that definition, the leader doesn't necessarily need to be the CEO. You do need to be able to obtain buy in and provide the resources, the authority, and I guess the space needed to achieve those goals together. As I said, I think that's going to be a definition that's going to be personalized, depending on who you ask.

Bill: Thank you for sharing that definition Alan. Your credentials are incredible. You lead the National Rural Health Association as it's CEO. You're recognized as being a top one hundred most influential people in healthcare. Talk about your journey and how you go to where you are as an expert in the healthcare space, particularly the rural healthcare space.

Alan: Yeah. Good question. In hindsight, to me looking back on my career so far, it seems to be a fairly straight and coherent path. It's funny how for anyone as you go through life, you have expectations and you go ahead, and how those things turn out vary from individual to individual. For me, it began in the state of Kansas, working in the governor's office. I began working in the constituents' services department dealing with Medicaid issues. After that I moved to Washington DC, I worked on Capitol Hill for a member of congress. Once again I was handling health care issues, but this time it was from the Medicare perspective. Then I spent ten years as a health care lobbyist here in our nation's capital, transitioning over to the National Rural Health Association. As I said, in hindsight it's a fairly straight path, twenty-six years dedicated towards health policy. I feel very fortunate that I've really found the area that I feel passionate about, and that's rural health.

Bill: Speaking of that, why the focus on rural health?

Alan: Rural health as a career path chose me more than I chose it. I'm from a one stoplight, or what used to be a one stoplight town in northeast Kansas, Holton, Kansas. I think most people tend to gravitate towards what they feel comfortable with and what they know. For me, that has always been a small town rural lifestyle. Going through the policy component, I certainly have been attracted to the health aspect of it. For me, it's just been a wonderful fit landing at the National Rural Health Association. I am fortunate to be able to focus in on a topic I passionately care about. That's been extremely beneficial for me personally.

Bill: Yes, passion can be a great motivator. Thank you because I know you've done a lot in the area of policy making and all that. You know it takes a lot to stay on top of all the complexities taking place in healthcare and rural health today. What would you say is your top leadership strength?

Alan: That certainly is the case with rural health. I think people that are not engaged in health policy or in particular rural health, you think rural and you default to say, "Well that's a small version of urban." It is not. It is a unique healthcare delivery environment.

Bill: Yes.

Alan: It's painful and complex. You talk about the different payment methodologies and challenges that go along with providing services in that context. I've got to tell you, for me personally, I would have to say collaboration and the ability to collaborate has been one of my strengths that has certainly carried me through in this role. You hear that all the time, I think, when people say, "Oh, the necessity to collaborate." In a rural context and certainly in a small organizational context, the ability to work with people who have different goals, different objectives, and in many cases, let's be honest, may not personally get along with you, and be able to collaborate for a greater good. That is such an important aspect to have and a necessity in this line of work.

Bill: Absolutely, and collaboration is one of those things that easier said than done, that's for sure.

Alan: Absolutely.

Bill: You've been the CEO for NRHA for the last eleven and a half years, coming up on twelve years now. What has been your biggest leadership challenge as the CEO of NRHA?

Alan: At NRHA, that can be summed up in the issue of direction and focus. There is one area that being the CEO of NRHA I have in common with a lot of CEOs of small rural hospitals or community health centers, being able to have a very diverse membership, constituency, and maintaining a clear-cut direction and focus for the organization going ahead. It's one of the greatest challenges. You can be taken a million different ways and being able to establish what's the end game, what are we trying to achieve here, that's ultimately important.

Bill: Yes. Based on what you're telling me, we just spoke briefly a few minutes ago about the complexity of rural health. I would guess as being the CEO of NRHA, it is complexity on steroids more or less.

Alan: Well it certainly is. Our membership includes clinicians, all sorts of physicians, allied health professionals, rural researchers, state employees that oversee rural programs. The breadth of policy interests that go into rural health are quite diverse. It is so difficult to maintain that common focus towards improving the health of rural communities, and keeping everyone aligned with the correct direction for the organization. It's an ongoing challenge.

Bill: Yes, I would think so. What do you see as the top issues that rural health leaders face today?

Alan: Well, it's kind of good news, bad news. The good news is, it's certainly an interesting time. The bad news is, it's a very interesting time. The healthcare system is changing dramatically. For rural leaders, the constant threat of being trampled underfoot by much larger health systems is a huge issue right now. The issues of workforce recruitment or retention and then put on top of that the financial challenges, that leaders are facing. It makes it a very, very difficult time for leaders to stay on top of the changing environment, and to make sure that their communities are positioned correctly as they move forward. Again I go back, what's the good news of that? I think there's tremendous opportunity for enhancement and growth, of moving ahead. It's certainly a challenging time, to say the least.

Bill: Yes. I mean I think if you ask any young person in high school what do you want to do when you get out of college, I don't think many of them would say, "I want to work for an organization where costs are rising, reimbursement is decreasing, and the complexity is overwhelming." There are a lot of issues we currently face.

Alan: That certainly is the case. The ironic part about that, at least from my perspective, is we face such challenges on workforce recruitment and retention. Anytime we get together and we talk about rural health policy and delivering rural health services, what do we mention? We mention all the challenges, and the problems we face, and the limited resources. Then it seems like we're dumbfounded that we have a hard time recruiting young professionals into these communities that we just told is a challenging environment to operate within.

Bill: Yes. I know that there was that report that came out earlier this year citing basically one in three rural hospitals are at risk of closure, which is going back to your good news, bad news message. That is bad that one in three rural hospitals are at risk, but the good news part of that is that two out of three hospitals are doing okay.

Alan: You're absolutely right on that. Again, the ones that are surviving and thriving in this environment are the ones that are taking an innovative approach to recruitment retention. They're engaging in Telehealth applications as well. They're finding business partners to collaborate with. There are certainly success stories to be found in this environment.

Bill: Well I like to focus on leadership, so those all sound like issues of leadership, finding and recruiting, engaging with others, finding business partners. You see a lot of leaders in the rural health area, a lot of rural hospital CEOs, that sort of thing. Are there common traits that you see among rural health leaders? If you do, what are they?

Alan: I wish there was a more complicated answer to this. This may be an over simplistic response to that. The one common trait I see among successful rural CEOs is quite simply, they are people people. They have the ability to navigate the politics of a small local community. Sometimes larger organizational CEOs are shielded away from the politics that you have in a local community. In a rural community, you have a board that sees you in the morning at the local restaurant. They'll see you during the day, and will see you at night at ball games, or at the grocery store. The ability to negotiate the local community politics and to be able to resonate well with people, it's a common trait that I believe rural leaders have, a unique skill set that they have to have in order to survive.

Bill: Well it is true. In the smaller communities, everybody knows everyone. That goes a long way. My dad was a minister, a country preacher, where I grew up. I couldn't get away with anything as a kid.

Alan: That is the rural experience, is it not?

Bill: Alan, you've seen a lot in your almost twelve years as a CEO at NRHA. What is your proudest moment as a CEO of NRHA so far?

Alan: Well, there's a lot that I can be proud of at NRHA, and everything that the organization has accomplished through that time. I've got to tell you, I personally feel like within the last year, from the CEO perspective, there are two proud moments I've had within the organization. First was when our senior vice-president of membership services, Brock Slabach, was awarded the Calico Leadership award by the National Rural Health Resource Center, earlier this year. Then that was followed up just last month by Amy Allezondo, who is our VP of program services, who was actually awarded the Texas A & M Department of Public Health

Outstanding Alumni of the year award. I think, as a CEO, your responsibility is to your team. How can you enable them or create an environment that they can achieve great things?

Brock and Amy certainly have achieved amazing things here at NRHA. Brock is leading the national discussion on quality improvement and alternative payment models. Amy is busy trying to launch a national community health worker program. The ability to be able to provide that context, that environment, and that space where your team members can be recognized nationally for their leadership roles, what greater accomplishment can anyone have as a leader than to see people, your peers achieving great things?

Bill: Well I very much appreciate that in your answer to your proudest moment as CEO. You are talking about two of the people that you work with instead of a narcissistic type answer that you could have given. It interestingly takes us back to how you defined leadership. When you gave us your definition of leadership, you talked about achieving common goals and helping others achieve those goals. Hats off to you for living your definition of leadership Alan.

Can you share anything with us, any stories or experiences that you've had, where you've seen a rural health leader do something unique that worked or that paid off?

Alan: There are so many examples of that. That is not surprising because NRHA, if you're a rural health leader, you're going to join the NRHA. Over the years, I've just seen so many different examples of that. I hate to pick one, but I will pick an amazing and funny story. Last year I was speaking to the Georgetown Health Policy class, talking about rural health and rural health policy. One of the students had asked if I had by chance heard of an innovative approach to workforce recruitment and retention, that was happening in rural America by a rural hospital CEO, that was actually providing international sabbaticals for his clinical staff. I interjected right then, and I said, "Yeah, yeah, yeah. That's Benjamin Anderson. He's from Kearny County Hospital in Lakin, Kansas." I said, "I talk with him almost weekly it seems like. He's busy changing the world of recruitment retention from the middle of nowhere in western Kansas."

I love the story of Benjamin because it really highlights the fact that it doesn't matter where you're located, you have the ability to be recognized and to change the health care delivery system nationally, just by being innovative and being a rural health leader. It struck me as funny, that I was here talking in DC at Georgetown University, and they were bringing up the name Benjamin Anderson. To me that's a unique perspective of how he's doing it. That is really made a big splash.

Bill: Interesting. Is he doing that for primarily for physicians?

Alan: Primarily for physicians. As you might imagine, western Kansas, that's a tough sell to get a clinician out there. If you've had the chance to drive through there, it is sparse. Many of those counties are designated as frontier counties. His pitch is come work for me, I'll give you the opportunity to actually practice your medicine internationally on a sabbatical. It's a tremendous recruitment approach.

Bill: Absolutely. I've heard about that myself. Thanks for sharing that.

In your opinion Alan, what do you think rural health leaders should be doing differently?

Alan: That is a tough question. It's a tough question because for most rural health professionals, it's one of the toughest gigs on the planet to have. I'm cautious in saying this. I really honestly believe that what attracts people to rural towns, is good education and good healthcare. I don't get a sense that nationally rural health leaders and most particularly rural hospital CEOs, are really treating their facility as the community asset that it is. The communication component of it, working and collaboration with local media to really highlight the role and importance of local healthcare, and maintaining that asset. It is a community asset. I think not doing that job adequately leads towards out-migration of patients, out of your community. Everything else flows, when you've got the community as a partner in delivering healthcare.

Bill: In the small town where I grew up, there were mixed feelings about our little rural hospital in our county there. Some people would drive right by it going to the bigger cities. I know it saved both of my parent's lives. It probably saved my brother's life for some of the ways I tortured him as a kid. Many of us in the community took it for granted.

I was talking to a CEO of a rural hospital here in Florida a few months ago. He impressed me so much when he said that he considers rural health as the gateway to world class medicine. That kind of goes along with what you're saying. It's truly an asset, and it truly can be a gateway to world class medicine or world class healthcare, however you want to say that.

Alan: Oh absolutely! I think it's one of the misnomers that people have that somehow rural healthcare is less than. Just looking at the national quality data, outcomes, and metrics for primary care, rural is as good and often times better than urban care for all the obvious reasons. Being able to share that information with your community is so very important.

Bill: Absolutely.

Alan, talk a little bit about the future of rural health as you see it.

Alan: Well, as I mentioned earlier, the entire healthcare system is changing dramatically. I just don't see how rural doesn't change with it. In fact, if you're looking for what are the innovative solutions in healthcare today, most things are happening in a rural context. The use of Telehealth, both eICU, Teleconsultation, Telepsych and Teleradiology are being pioneered in rural settings. New and innovative approaches to utilize technology by all healthcare practitioners, not just rural, is having an impact everywhere. Rural health is taking the lead in moving towards the focus on primary care, ensuring that rural communities focus on their health of their community and not just the health once they show up at the hospital. That's going to be key as well. There are a lot of innovative approaches that we're seeing. I think those are going to continue with a much stronger focus on keeping people healthy and out of the hospital to begin with.

Bill: Very much health population, health management type concepts.

Alan: Absolutely.

Bill: What scares you the most about the future of rural health Alan?

Alan: That's a tough one to answer. Historically, health care in rural communities have survived and thrived because it has been a community focus. Communities have directed where they want their healthcare system to go. You see from the board of trustees' approach in rural hospitals or rural community health centers to how clinicians engage in the community. With the changing nature of our healthcare system, I'm really worried that there's such a focus on volume and efficiency, that it's driving the system to much larger ownership control outside of the community. Obviously, the worrisome note in that is, if you're making decisions based solely on efficiency and finance from those that are not living within the community, you have a real potential to remove that healthcare access from the community.

You have to potentially change rural America going ahead in the next five to ten years. That ties into this rural hospital closure crisis that we're seeing. I think when you look at the national data, more people are moving towards rural than they have in the past. That's showing through the census estimates. We just need to make sure that rural is a place for those that want to have that lifestyle, that they can continue to have that lifestyle going ahead. There's a real concern with the changing business of healthcare, that rural may be left behind.

Bill: That's what scares you. You've already talked a little bit about what excites you, but what excites you the most about the future?

Alan: Oh, I think just the opportunity to focus in on keeping people healthy in the community. I can't say that enough. Look at the national data. Unfortunately, since 1991 until today, we started to see life expectancy diverge. People in urban areas are living longer than those in rural. In fact, in the most rural communities, you are seeing the life expectancy actually decrease. There's got to be a focus on the community in keeping people healthy, and promoting healthy lifestyles and healthy choices. That does excite me, that we have this national direction. Hopefully rural leaders can take advantage of this going ahead, and we can see some dramatic improvements in rural healthcare status for these communities.

Bill: I was just reading an article last week, and I saw your name with a quote from you. You were talking about obesity in rural America, and some of the challenges that rural hospitals and rural healthcare providers face, and how they're dealing with that.

Alan: It is a tough situation. The communities act as communities act. When you've got a community that's not focused in on healthy lifestyle choices, you've just got a spiraling effect of that as well. To the credit of healthcare providers, we've got to find a new reimbursement system that actually adequately provides compensation to keep the community healthy. Our current reimbursement model pays when people are sick. That is a transformation that has to happen. I think you're starting to see those inroads made across the U.S. We're certainly hopeful they continue going ahead.

Bill: We've covered a lot of ground so far in our conversation, Alan. I have one last question for you. If there's only one nugget of information that everybody takes away from our conversation, what should that be?

Alan: The necessity for collaboration and leadership. The ability to work with people that you may not necessarily agree with, to achieve the goals that you need to achieve. That is a lesson that I've seen successful rural health leaders employ. It's something that not only should be advanced in rural, it's something that urban CEOs certainly can learn from their rural counterparts as well too.

Bill: Absolutely.

Alan: The need to collaborate for the greater goal.

Bill: Well said Alan! Thank you again for joining us today Alan and for sharing your knowledge and expertise about rural health.

R.D. Williams

Episode five of Rural Health Leadership Radio is an interview with the CEO of Hendry Regional Medical Center, R.D. Williams. As we discuss the ups and downs of leadership, as well as how Williams inspired me to create Rural Health Leadership Radio, we touch on important ways to improve rural healthcare, as well as some ways that didn't work out so well. Topics such as maximizing financial resources, knowing and anticipating community needs, recruiting the correct types of physicians for the community, and many others are discussed during our interview.

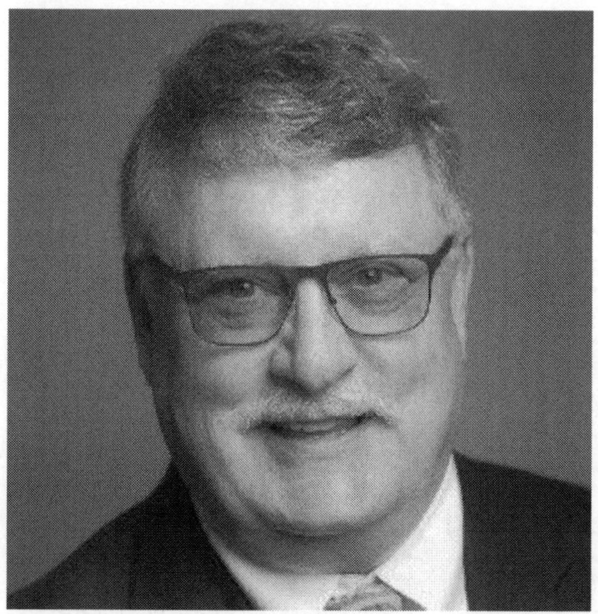

Bill: R.D. is celebrating his 3-year anniversary as the CEO at Hendry Regional Medical Center, having started in June of 2013.

Prior to that, he was the CEO at Ashe Memorial Hospital in Jefferson, North Carolina, for around 19 years, starting in November of '94 until May of 2013. He received his undergraduate degree at the Medical College of Virginia with a B.S. in healthcare management in 1981, and then earned his MBA at the Virginia Commonwealth University in 1986.

He's worked in a variety of hospitals in Texas, Oklahoma, Kentucky, Tennessee, North Carolina, Virginia, and now in Florida. You get around, R.D.

RD: I try to.

Bill: R.D. is originally from Roanoke, Virginia, and he's certainly involved in the community. He's a member of the Clewiston Rotary Club; he serves as the Clewiston Chamber of Commerce President; he serves on the Hendry County Economic Development Council, and also as the Chair of the

Administrative Council at the Clewiston First United Methodist Church.

He enjoys playing golf, reading, home restoration, and working on his 1973 MGB automobile. I always wanted one of those MGBs. I loved the rounded corners of those. He's married to LuAnn with 3 adult sons and 2 granddaughters, ages 9 and 2.

I certainly appreciate you joining us, RD, because you were the inspiration for creating this podcast. At the time you didn't realize it, but you and I were having a conversation last year and I asked you about one of the challenges of being a CEO of a rural hospital. You told me that it's hard to find out what other rural health leaders are doing at their respective hospitals because there is not a great sharing of information.

The only way you could realize and learn what other rural health leaders were doing was by spending time and money by traveling to meetings, but you didn't always have time and money. After we had that conversation, I was actually listening to one of my favorite podcasts when a light bulb went off. I thought to myself, "Hey, I should start a podcast to help R.D. and all the other rural health CEOs and leaders out there." Thank you for that inspiration!

RD: Well, I'm happy to be what help I can.

Bill: Let me ask you this: You've had a lot of experience in healthcare, why did you choose healthcare as an occupation to begin with?

RD: You know, Bill, sometimes I think I didn't have a choice, but obviously I did. My father was a hospital administrator in Roanoke, Virginia at Roanoke Memorial Hospital for over 32 years. My mother is a nursing educator. She taught in the health careers program at Patrick Henry Hospital and some other nursing programs throughout her career. It was dinner table conversation for as long as I can remember.

Bill: It's in your DNA?

RD: You could say that, yes.

Bill: Did you consider other industries for a career or was it no question, healthcare was your career path?

RD: Well, when I finally realized that I would not be successful playing professional football at 5'11", 240, I decided once I came down to reality I decided to work in a career that I thought I could make a difference for other people. It's really what a lot of folks are in healthcare for, it's because they can make a difference in other folks' lives and improve the community.

I was able to follow through with it and I've been fortunate to work for some good companies and some good hospitals, and working with great groups of people at each organization to be able to accomplish those goals.

Bill: I appreciate what you just said about serving the community and everything. Obviously in addition to being the CEO of a hospital, you serve your community with all the activities you're involved in. I don't see how you have time to play golf, though, or read or do home restoration, or even drive that MGB, let alone work on it.

RD: Well, you make time. It's all in how you want to spend your time.

Bill: You chose healthcare as a career path. Why rural heath?

RD: Well, I've worked in urban hospitals and rural hospitals. While I enjoyed my stay in the urban hospitals in Richmond, Virginia, Charlotte, North Carolina and Louisville, Kentucky, I really enjoyed my work in rural communities. One, Roanoke, even though it's a metropolitan area, it is a small town. It's a small town of 200,000 people, but it's a much smaller town with how the relationships are among people and neighborhoods. I really enjoyed that. I wanted to raise my children in that type of atmosphere and give them the same type of opportunities that I had to understand what their community was and be a part of it.

In rural healthcare, or in rural hospitals, many times you're the major employer in the community. You're an employer of choice. You can really have an impact on the entire community, and how well you do your job or how poorly you do your job is reflected very quickly within the community. I just like being able to have that impact and to see what's going on in the community around me and know that by doing a good job we're impacting my neighbors' and friends' lives.

Bill: That's an important responsibility.

I have to admit that I'm a leadership nerd. Nerds usually like to collect unusual things and I like to collect definitions of leadership. They're easy to store and you don't have to dust them. I'm looking to add to my collection so, how do you define leadership?

RD: I look at leadership as being able to pull a group of people together, decide upon some common goals in a common direction for the organization to be able to facilitate moving forward in that direction. I don't believe leadership is doing everything yourself, but being able to empower and engage the people you work with to achieving that common goal that your organization has.

Bill: Empowerment, engagement. I like those words. I like putting those on the shelf of my leadership definition collection. I like what you said about deciding on common goals and pulling that group of people together. You have several key words in your definition that I like, and hopefully our listeners do too, so I appreciate your definition of leadership. When it comes to leadership, what would you say is your top leadership strength?

RD: I think my leadership style and leadership skills have evolved over time. I have found that listening to people is a skill that's very important and a skill that I've tried to cultivate over time. Also, a willingness to let others fail. It sounds a little odd, but I had some mentors as I was growing in the profession and they allowed me to try things and fail.

They might've known I was going to fail, but they knew that I had to learn those things myself. That made me a stronger leader and decision maker in the future. I want the folks that I work with to have the freedom to try things, to innovate, and just knowing that sometimes not everything you try to do is going to be successful.

Bill: That is an interesting concept. Very interesting. A willingness to let others fail. Can you provide an example from your own personal experience or someone that you worked with where you've done that? We all fear failure from one degree or another and the consequences of that. How do you know when to let someone do that? Do you have to determine what the consequences might be? How do you do that?

RD: You are working for a common set of goals within your organization and moving your organization towards achieving those goals. Different folks that you work with have different passions and different interests. I know that I've worked in some communities where a number of folks felt like we needed a particular type of physician in the community. We set out and recruited those folks and set them up, and it didn't work. It failed. The practice didn't thrive.

It was either we didn't know enough to support the individual or the individual, once they got there, decided that the rural life and the rural lifestyle, the responsibilities of being a one of a kind in the community, just didn't work for them.

That helped me learn how to bring in physicians or bring in providers, specialties, or other services in the community and to know and anticipate some of the problems that may occur in the future as we were trying to develop some programs like that in a rural community.

Bill: Thank you. The other thing you mentioned is listening. That sounds like that's something that you've worked on intentionally, to be a better listener.

RD: Well, it was. I hate to say it's been a more recent innovation or acquired skill for me. I had the opportunity back in the early 2000s to participate in a lean collaborative among 5 hospitals making a transformational change in leadership in those organizations.

What I found as we went through the process of applying the lean techniques to healthcare was that you've got to listen to the people that are doing the work. They're the ones that know how to make improvements and know to make changes and ultimately impact the outcome for the customer or for the patient.

I found out very quickly that I didn't know everything. I might've thought I knew everything at one time or another, but I've been humbled more than once. I find it's quicker for me to listen to other people's ideas.

Bill: Absolutely.

RD: Let them try it.

Bill: Sure! You know, it's interesting. Listening is obviously a critical component of being an effective communicator. I've done, and other people have done, surveys of leaders. Generally speaking, of course, when you make a general statement like I'm about to make you can always shoot holes in it, but most leaders feel like they're great communicators. Regardless of which specific skill of communication you're talking about, most leaders feel like they're great communicators.

When you survey their constituents, the constituents usually say that they wish their leaders were better communicators. We're always fighting that battle of communication, trying to be more effective communicators, but it's certainly an integral part of leadership. I applaud you for what you shared about listening.

R.D. is also the inspiration of Rural Health Leadership Radio, and I thank you for that, R.D.

RD: Well, I really appreciate that, the opportunity to speak with you. I know you have ideas about how you wanted to communicate with folks, so I'm sure I wasn't the total genesis of that.

Bill: Well, I've given you credit so please take it.

RD: Okay.

Bill: You've shared a lot of great stuff so far, but talk about something unique that you've done as a rural health leader that worked.

RD: Many times, in rural communities, especially impoverished rural communities, which I seem to end up in, there're a number of health and human service providers throughout the community. Some of them might be in the private sector and some might be governmental, and some might be not for profit. Well, we're all faced with the same opportunity to serve a group of patients or a group of customers. We're charged with completing certain tasks and don't have necessarily all the financial resources to do those with.

We've been successful a couple of times in pulling groups of health and human service providers into a coalition or a coordinated effort to deliver care or deliver services throughout the communities that we serve in a way that reduces duplication and maximizes the use of the resources that we do have.

It allows us to apply for grant funding when they want coalitions of people coming together. Also, it allows us to work together to determine from the people that we serve what they actually need and tailor how we're all making offerings in the community to best fit the needs and the perceived needs of the folks that we're delivering services to.

It's got to be non-confrontational. No one in the group is looking for credit. It's not who put this together and who's had the greatest success or who's making or getting all the accolades for pulling it together. It's the group as a whole being able to impact the communities that we serve, the health of those communities, and the sustainability of the initiatives that we create.

Bill: That sounds like a lot of work. What are the challenges of coordinating all that? That seems very daunting, like a very daunting task.

RD: Initially it's a matter of developing trust among all the participants in the group. Yes, there's time involved. As you grow to know people within an organization it takes time. You've got to break bread with them. You've got to spend some time jointly coming together and doing that community health needs assessment or something equivalent to that. Deciding on a framework on how you can divide up the work and how you can support each other in your initiatives.

It's really just allowing each of those organizations to work smarter and to focus on a narrower scope of a problem, knowing that they've got other people that are focusing on other areas and together the missions of all our organizations are going to take place.

You have to have somebody coordinating those efforts. It might be an outreach coordinator at a hospital, or it might be a community advocate from the health department or one of the leaders of a charitable organization within the community. Somebody that's got a passion and a vision that if we can go from A to B, the health of our community's going to be so much better.

Bill: That sounds like a great example of your definition of leadership because your definition talked about pulling a group of people together to move forward towards common goals, empowering them and engaging them. It's a living example of your definition of leadership. I love that.

RD: Well, thank you.

Bill: Everyone likes to talk about something they've done that's worked, but we can learn just as much, sometimes even more, by talking about something that we've tried that didn't necessarily work or didn't turn out the way we'd planned. Can you talk about something that you've tried that didn't work out the way you'd planned?

RD: I started in the facility in North Carolina in 1994. Something that's real commonplace right now in hospitals throughout the country is a tobacco free environment. Well, you know, when that was happening in the early, mid 2000s, there was a lot of angst and controversy among a lot of the public, but consider taking a hospital in the number 1 tobacco producing state in the country trying to do a tobacco free status in 1996 before anybody else had done it.

It was the right thing to do and it was a great initiative. I learned a tremendous new vocabulary. It's not the words that were new, but it's the combination of those words. Being called just all kinds of interesting things except a nice person. It was the right thing to do, but it failed.

Eventually the time for that came around 6 or 8 years later. There was a statewide initiative, a national initiative, to go to tobacco free on all your healthcare campuses, and we did it then.

Bill: Good.

RD: We're able to be successful and sustain it.

Bill: You like challenges.

RD: Yes, we can't be afraid of a challenge.

Bill: That's true, and timing is everything. Thank you for sharing that with us. In your opinion, R.D., you've been around, you've seen a lot of things in your career. What do you think rural health leaders need to do differently?

RD: You really can't be a specialist. You've got to be a generalist. You've got to wear many hats. You have to be willing to understand and be able to support folks at all levels of the organization. You've got to keep up with employee relations and physician relations and employee development, board development. Everything that's going on in the community.

You have to have a firm understanding of finances because you can have the greatest quality organization around and perfect customer satisfaction, but if you're not billing and collecting for the things that you provide you're not going to be able to sustain those services.

Many times, in a rural organization you just don't have the depth in the organization that you might have in a more urban area nor the specialization like many of the large facilities do. I think you got to wear all those many hats, and you've definitely got to be engaged in the community and engaged with your workforce because you've got to have that. Win their hearts and minds if you're going to be successful in competing with the bright lights and big cities down the road that are trying to siphon off your patients.

Bill: That seems to be a challenge for everybody. With 1 out of 3 rural hospitals at risk of closing, it's a tall order. We've got our work cut out for us. Well, I'm going to ask you 2 more questions. You can answer in whatever order you want because they're basically the same question, just from different perspectives. My two questions are, what excites you the most about the future, and the opposite of that, what scares you the most about the future?

RD: What excites me the most about the future, especially in healthcare, there's just tremendous opportunity, especially in the rural organizations as technology changes. It's exciting to be able to expand the services and improve the care that we deliver to the communities we serve. Many of our communities have the same profile. They're poor, they're old, they lack transportation. Because of that, they don't necessarily have access to the different services that improve their quality of life.

As technology improves and we're able to bring technology to bear and just wisely decide how we're going to deliver care, we can have that dramatic impact and make an improvement in the quality of life in the communities that we serve.

What scares me the most is the ability to be able to provide those changes in technology. It comes at a price. The price very often is financially-driven. It's not just the human cost and those types of things. We've got to have money to be able to provide these services. As I mentioned, most of our communities are impoverished. They don't have disposable assets to make that co-payment or meet that deductible. We have to be able to operate much leaner and do the right things.

I see the changes in the federal and state reimbursement programs and the commercial insurance programs that are making it tougher and tougher for rural organizations, small organizations, to be able to survive. Government payers say, "Well, here's the plan." You know you've got 50,000 people to serve. It should only take you $1,000 a person to do that. Well, if you're serving a million people and you get $1,000 a person, that's a lot different than 50,000 with $1,000 a person.

I think what scares me is that the payment reforms and the pressure to reduce costs and to make things tighter and tighter are going to continue to drive down access to care in rural communities, especially as more and more organizations close or have to change the way they deliver services in those communities.

Bill: Thank you for sharing that perspective. Any last word from you, R.D., that you want to share, or do you have it all out there?

RD: I'm sure we could talk for hours if we wanted to, Bill.

Bill: That's true.

RD: I really appreciate the opportunity. I think that, as you've said, I mentioned, that I don't have a lot of opportunity to get out and network with people on a face-to-face basis. I think being able to listen to people's ideas and experiences in a format like this will be very helpful.

Bill: Thank you and thank you for your inspiration. I appreciate your humility on that as well, so thank you, RD. Thank you for inspiring me to do this and thank you for sharing your thoughts, your experiences, and your outlook on rural health.

Brock Slabach

In this interview with Senior Vice President for the Member Services at the National Rural Health Association, Brock Slabach, a variety of rural health topics are considered. Brock discusses, in detail, the three items he believes have the biggest impact on rural health: identity, information, and relationships. We also look at how making mistakes and learning from them improves the success of a health leader, as well as the impact of the rapid change in rural health care along with the importance of innovation. Furthermore, we discuss Brock's work on the Save Rural Hospitals Act and more.

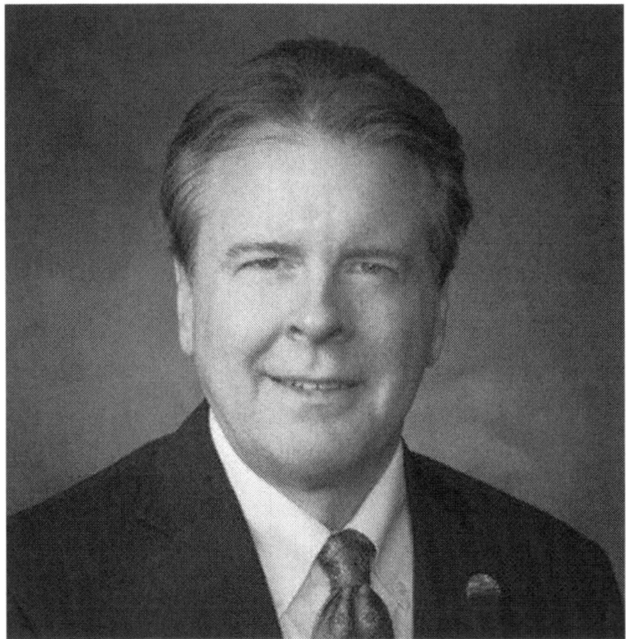

Bill: Brock Slabach is currently serving as the Senior Vice President of Member Services for the National Rural Health Association (NRHA). The NRHA is a membership organization with over 21,000 members nationwide. Brock has over 28 years of experience in administration of rural hospitals. For 20 years, from 1987 through 2007, he was the Administrator of Field Memorial Community Hospital in Centreville, Mississippi. Brock earned his Bachelor of Science from Oklahoma Baptist University, and his Master of Public Health in Health Administration from the University of Oklahoma. I'm guessing you might have grown up in Oklahoma.

Brock: I grew up in southern Kansas, as a matter of fact.

Bill: Southern Kansas! Okay! Thank you for joining us today Brock. I appreciate you taking time out of your busy schedule. I've had the opportunity to listen to you speak in front of groups on more than one occasion, and your breadth of knowledge and expertise, when it comes to leadership in rural health, is incredible, so thank you for being here.

Brock: You're welcome.

Bill: I've got several questions I want to ask you, so let's get going.

Brock: Sure.

Bill: When we choose our career paths in life, there are all kinds of industries we can choose from. Why did you choose healthcare as an occupation?

Brock: That's a good question. I guess it found me. Right out of high school, I went to college and began working in Respiratory Therapy at a hospital. That was at about the age of 19. Then after that, I went to graduate school at the University of Oklahoma, as you mentioned, and I didn't have any consideration for anything other than healthcare.

Bill: Why rural health?

Brock: I grew up in rural Kansas. I appreciate the values of individuals that live there. I think that we have to be very conscious of the fact that all of the energy that it takes to run this country, in terms of energy related to petroleum, to all of the crops that feed us, are very important to the economy of these United States. My family, going back several generations on both sides, has been farmers in Kansas. This has been our life's work. It's my strong belief that individuals in rural areas, regardless of their geography, should have access to quality healthcare. That became kind of a mission for me, and it was expressed through my delight to have served in rural hospitals in several parts of the United States, most recently in Mississippi.

Bill: Twenty years as a CEO of any hospital is quite a record. Hospital CEO turnover is rather high these days. Twenty years at the same facility is quite impressive. How did you do that?

Brock: For a hospital administrator, you look for several factors that will play very much into your ability to do a good job. I was blessed to have had the crucible of those factors that really served to help me to have a wonderful career at that facility. There are three factors that I learned in graduate school. It's the medical staff, the board, and then the community or the hospital itself. Those three, that three-legged stool, if you will, made for a tremendous opportunity for me to exercise some of the gifts that I had, make mistakes, learn from those mistakes, and reapply the learning into, hopefully, something better. It was a great experience, and it's a place that is still going well. I'm pleased to see that they've done a great job with the work they're doing in that facility since I left.

Bill: I admit this regularly: I am a leadership nerd. I like to collect definitions of leadership and I'm looking to add to my collection. How do you define leadership?

Brock: Leadership, I guess classically, is just the ability to lead others. I'd distinguish that, definitely, from what I would call management, which I think is using very quantitative sorts of analysis to be able to achieve an outcome. Leadership is much more subjective, so it's not as easily defined. I like to say, like other things, you know it when you see it. I also believe, and I've come to learn, that leadership is a skill that's acquired, not necessarily taught. I think that you could learn some of the rubrics of leadership, but then some people just seem to have it and some people don't. I think that's part of the discernment that we go through in our jobs and in our careers, trying to decide where we best fit in terms of that analysis.

Bill: Thank you. I'm happy to add that to my collection. What would you say, Brock, is your top leadership strength?

Brock: It's my ability to see the big picture, taking disparate pieces of a puzzle, if you will, and beginning to see a pattern that exists beyond what's just readily recognizable on the surface. I think that leaders are good at being able to take what may seem amorphous or appear irregular or chaotic, and see order within that chaos, to begin to interpreting that in a different fashion for those that are following, so that they can see a vision of something well beyond themselves.

Bill: That's interesting. I like the saying, "Gaining clarity from chaos." That's a great strength to have. If you're the CEO of a rural hospital, you get to do that a lot.

Brock: That is one of the traits that I think are important for a rural hospital administrator, indeed.

Bill: Brock, you've been a hospital CEO, and now, in your role as Senior VP for Member Services at NRHA, you see and deal with a lot of leaders in rural health. You see a lot of things that are going on in rural health. Can you share some of the trends you are currently seeing that are having an impact on rural hospitals?

Brock: Sure. I think that more-so than any time in my career, there is a rapid progression of change that is just becoming more innovative all the time. I'm saying something that anybody initiated into this industry now will appreciate. I think that this change is creating the need for innovation, an innovation that is going to be relevant to our operations in rural hospitals to take us into a path that is different than maybe what we would've thought before. I think rural leaders have to take the chaos that's being given to us and really inquire into three basic areas of their organizations and look to see how that then comes out in the end in terms of planning.

The first is identity, basically asking, "Who are we? What are we here for? What is our mission?" That may change based on some of the dynamics of healthcare. Over the last twenty years, we've seen a decrease in the inpatient days of our facilities. We're becoming much more outpatient centered. The treatment plans for patients now require so much less need for classic inpatient or extended stays, so there's a tremendous change in technology that's helped to improve the situation.

Medications have improved so that many medications can be taken on an outpatient basis at home. You don't have to be hospitalized for some of those things anymore. We have to look at our identity. What are we? Who are we? Who are the people that we're serving? What are their needs, based on a community health needs assessment? That really takes into account what the community may benefit from, not from an institutional point of view, but what is it that the people, the folks that you're serving, really need to affect the health or the status of the population?

The second thing a leader could do is look at information. How does information flow within and outside of the organization? Is it bottled up and kept neatly in just one specific place, or is it being shared freely among all individuals that have a need to know? I think part of the problem in our society, and in our organizations, is that it's difficult to communicate the information that's necessary for everyone to know their job, number one. Number two, how do they fit into that bigger picture? How do they fit into the overall theme or mission about what the organization is for?

Last, and I think this is perhaps the most important one: how does a rural hospital administrator foster relationships? Relationships are the key, I think, in terms of the ability for them to do their jobs effectively. In relationships I'm talking about now, that white space on the organizational chart. I look at the quality. I can tell you today that if I go into a hospital, I can say that the quality of that organization's medical practice, or their quality of the hospital services they provide, is directly proportional to the quality of the relationships that exist within that organization.

Good leaders go about fostering those relationships and know how to facilitate process so that issues are tended to quickly and dealt with in an effective fashion. I look at identity, information, and relationships as being three key characteristics of a leader that really creates, I think, what it takes to produce a really top-notch quality facility.

Bill: I love that Brock. The succinct three bullet points: identity, information, and relationships. While you're referring to information as internal to the organization, I mean the whole idea behind this podcast was a conversation I was having with the CEO of a critical access hospital in Florida when I asked him about what were some of the challenges he faced. He was sharing with me that it's not always easy to know what a CEO at another rural hospital is doing, what's working, what's not working, the sharing of information between hospitals.

He said, "I can spend time and money to travel to and attend a meeting where there is great sharing of information, but I can't always get away to go to those meetings." That's why this podcast was created, to help share information like you're sharing with us here amongst hospital CEOs and other rural health leaders, to help us all be a rising tide that lifts all ships in rural health. Thank you. I like your conciseness as well.

I love the information that you're sharing with us Brock.

Are you ready to keep rolling here?

Brock: I sure am.

Bill: In your role, you hear a lot of conversations and what's going on about policy that's taking place, policy that's being developed to solve some of the challenges that rural health leaders face. What are some of the observations you've made of late about those policy considerations that are being developed?

Brock: We are responding to the challenges I mentioned in the previous segment by looking at how rural communities can transform their healthcare services to be more responsive to community need. We're looking at the unfortunate event of rural hospital closures. We've had 75 since 2010, and that number appears to be growing. This year, we're so far at 15 rural hospital closures. No, I'm sorry, 12. We've had 18 during the entirety of 2015, so we're seeing transitions happen, whether they're desired or not, in rural communities. We've been able to partner with representatives, Sam Graves and Dave Loebsack, from Missouri and Iowa respectively. We put forward House Resolution 3225, known as the Save Rural Hospitals Act, which really addresses a lot of the key areas of what's negatively impacting rural hospitals today.

The first is reimbursement levels due to sequestration, that's the 2% reduction in all Medicare payments. Then the reduction in the bad-debt allowance for Medicare patients from 100% down to 65%. Those 2 policy features have seriously eroded the ability for rural hospitals to be able to serve their communities effectively. This Save Rural Hospitals Act, for example, reverses the 2% to sequestration and then also the 35% cut in bad-debt reimbursement.

More importantly, in addition to a number of other provisions, it allows for the introduction of a new provider type. We happen to call it the Community Outpatient Hospital. This is a new program that would be available to communities who really needed services that fit in between a clinic and a critical access hospital or small rural PPS hospital. This Community Outpatient Hospital would serve a community through a free-standing emergency department with the opportunity for observation status would be able to do population health activities and chronic care management through a clinic that may be attached to this unit, and all of that at 105% of cost with an additional wrap-around grant that's afforded in this particular piece of legislation. We think this could be a real important introduction to being responsive to community need through innovating our provider types or the facilities that are actually being implemented now.

The other part of this, Bill, is that it will seek to stabilize operations of all facilities and then offer a life-rope to those that need a new model in which to be able to serve the community that they're in.

Bill: Any prediction on The Save The Rural Hospital Act?

Brock: We're working in an environment now of complete dysfunction when it comes to congressional activity.

Bill: Nothing like an election year.

Brock: Yeah, and that complicates it even further. We're hoping that we can gain traction in both houses of the congress, and maybe when we come back next year, work really hard to try to get that passed. In the meantime, we have some significant problems that are happening. We just had hospitals that closed in Georgia and Tennessee recently, so I think obviously the timing of this is incredibly important. We have some pretty severe situations going on right now.

Our analysis shows that there's roughly 673 rural hospitals that are either at risk or at high-risk for closure right now. That's out of about 1,855 total numbers of rural hospitals, so that's a pretty significant number of those that are really experiencing stressful times right now.

Bill: Thank you for your work on that, and continued success on moving that forward. Can you tell something unique that you've observed, maybe you've done yourself as a rural health leader, or that you've seen another rural health leader try that worked. I think we need as many ideas as possible on how to keep our facilities open and serving our communities.

Brock: I've seen colleagues that have done just beautiful work in the area of relationships and being a crucible or fostering really strong relationships within the organization to produce a common good. I mentioned this earlier in one of the three points.

We need to be very intentional about creating facilities that can facilitate process. How do you actually create relationships that are effective? What I like to say is that we have technical individuals in our facilities that have really mastered a particular trade, let's say x-ray technician, a registered nurse, or a physician, but I've observed that, over time, many of these individuals may still be at the kindergarten level in terms of their ability to be able to get along with each other. A lot of times this isn't because they are bad people or that they don't intend to do well. It's just that they haven't learned techniques on how to be capable to relate to each other in a way that's productive. I think fostering relationships, being able to deal with that, and implement policies and procedures that help move that along.

Leaders that I've seen that do very well, including a physician at my hospital in Mississippi, did this beautifully, that is developing a clear identity that lights the dark in moments of confusion. Being able to take stressful times and communicate the fact that, "Gosh, we've been here before. This is not something that we're not used to." Go back to 1945 and give examples of what the organization has been through in terms of stresses and say that, "Look, this too we shall overcome." We can only do what we can to be able to help light the way for these moments of time when organizations, and all organizations can be stressed. Support employees through this process, not only employees but the community, being able to facilitate that kind of comprehension that goes beyond maybe just the facts and figures. I think that's an important element of what I see that's important for leaders that I've seen that I liked to try to emulate in terms of my practice.

Bill: Now I know why I like to listen to your presentations, Brock. You just dropped a pearl right into my lap that I wrote down. "Developing an identity that lights the dark in times of confusion." Beautiful!

Tell us about something that you've done or you've seen another rural health leader try that didn't work. We like to talk about our successes, but sometimes we can learn even more from trying something that didn't work or didn't turn out the way we planned.

Brock: That's another great question. I see lots of failed efforts at times, and those are certainly not happy, and hopefully they don't cost very much in terms of dollars, in terms of repair. I think that what I've seen most of the times that have led to problems for my colleagues is basically taking very complex situations and making or issuing very simple solutions. I like what Oscar Wilde said, "For every great problem there is a simple solution, and it's usually wrong." I think some problems do need to be broken down into its simplest components in order to solve it. That is the way we use those building blocks to deal with complexity. We deal with a lot of complex situations right now. Unfortunately, there're not many silver bullets that're going to correct the courses of many of our organizations. It's going to take the power of everybody coming together within the organization, and fostering the brilliance that everybody has, to be able to solve some of those issues.

Understanding complexity is essential to effective leadership. I'll never forget an experience I had where understanding complexity saved the day. I was told by somebody that came to my hospital that we could do a wound care program and make all kinds of money based on the billings for that service. Thank goodness I had some excellent coders in my coding department who stood their ground and said, "No, we can't bill that. Even though money would be great, this is not compliant with proper Medicare billing guidelines." I said, "Look, you're right. We can't do it," and we ended up doing the right thing. I didn't follow through with everything that I needed to in the beginning. I was a little bit short, but it all came out in the end because I had some great folks that I depended upon to guide me and correct the mistakes that I made in terms of some of my simple understanding of the situation.

Bill: That's great, because it's very tempting if you're under the impression that it could make a financial difference for your facility, but like you said, you've got to do what's right and depend on those with the expertise to help in that decision-making process.

Brock: Oh yeah, I was told by the folks that advised me, "Oh yeah, this is great. You can do it this way. No problem."

It didn't turn out that way.

Bill: Amazing!

Brock, what do you think that rural health leaders need to do differently?

Brock: It may be somewhat repetitive, but I think that looking at how innovation could become a central part to their operation, and looking at how innovations- when I talk about innovations now, I'm talking now in the bigger picture regarding alternative payment models, and then delivery system reform. Medicare, through Centers for Medicare and Medicaid Innovation have put forward, and they continue to put forward, all kinds of innovations regarding payment models. These are creating a whole different set of incentives for us in terms of how we do our business. It's almost turning upside down the industry that we're in. How do we translate those innovations into a rural context? I challenge everybody to make sure they tend to a couple of very important things.

First, if you're operating clinics, or if you have clinics associated with your hospital, make sure that they're looking at clinic care management, or CCM, as a billing source because now Medicare pays even in a rural health clinic for chronic care management. The other is taking advantage of the annual wellness visit, or AWV.

Medicare, several years ago, began paying for a benefit to everyone over 65 enrolled in Medicare to receive an annual wellness visit. I would encourage every listener to make sure that wherever they have the influence, that they're implementing chronic care management services using the program available, and then also doing annual wellness visits.

This is a step towards a patient centered medical home. You'll never go wrong in terms of moving your system or your services of your facility into a primary care medical home context. Those are some very basic building blocks to get there. That's an example of innovation that really needs to start to take root in local organizations. Trying to take current payment model introduction and then how can that be translated into a delivery system reform at the local level?

Bill: Excellent. Great information. With the state that rural health is in, as you said, one in three rural hospitals are at risk of closing, so a lot of scary stuff going on out there, but what excites you the most about the future?

Brock: Without a doubt, I've told friends and colleagues this; I remember sitting at my hospital years ago wondering if there's ever an end to this consistent cycle of viewing disease as billable services, and doing the same thing over and over and over again, and never getting any different result. We would just keep perpetuating the same sick care system that we've always had. I see an opportunity now that I would sit there in my chair as a hospital administrator, and say, "What if we moved upstream and treated disease differently? What if we looked at prevention and care management across a continuum more deliberately with payment incentives that would be able to help us to be able to achieve that?" I finally see a glimmer of where now this is starting to become the reality.

One of the saddest days in my community, when I was in Mississippi, was when a company came in and started a dialysis center for end-stage renal disease. I was at the ribbon cutting, and I was pleased, of course, that we had this service locally being offered through this company. Then it just dawned on me that this is a result, really, of bad policy in terms of being able to treat patients upstream better so that they don't have to end up on dialysis at some point. I finally see an opportunity for that to happen.

One of the reasons why I'm so passionate about where we are right now is, even though we have all this chaos, even though we have a lot of trouble, I do see a hope of something better that's coming in terms of a way that we can organize care around population health, and then being able to organize our communities in such a way to be able to achieve those goals. I do see a lot of optimism, and one of my goals is to be able to share that optimism as much as I can in the bigger picture with those that I have contact with.

Bill: You have done exactly that, Brock. You have proven what I said earlier, that you are a tremendous resource of knowledge and expertise when it comes to leadership in rural health. Thank you so much for sharing your experiences in rural health, your observations, your knowledge, and your expertise.

Kris Allen

Eaton Rapids Medical Center's Vice President of Patient Services, Kris Allen, discussed multiple rural health topics in our August 30, 2016 interview. She identifies collaboration and influence as two of the most important aspects of leadership, and it's seen in her responses throughout the interview. There is discussion of making healthcare more customer service oriented by being more proactive instead of reactive by doing things such as rounding, strategic planning three to five years in advance, and preparing for the breadth of legislative changes that are coming in rural healthcare. These, and many other topics, are dealt with in detail in our discussion with Kris Allen.

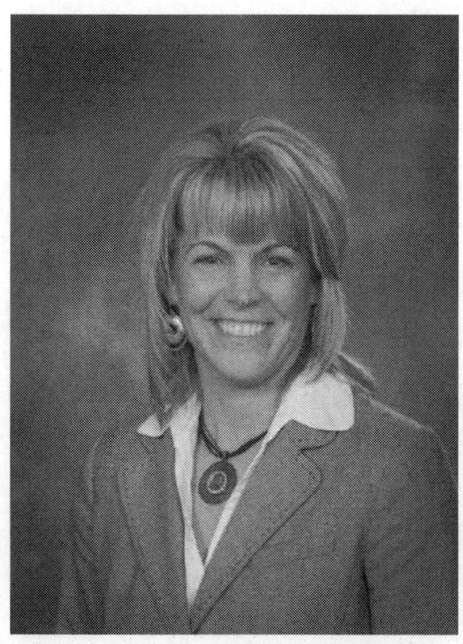

Bill: Kris Allen is the Vice President of Patient Services at Eaton Rapids Medical Center in Eaton Rapids, Michigan. She has been in healthcare for over 15 years as a registered nurse. Kris started her nursing career in the general and the medical inpatient area with a special focus on orthopedics. She quickly moved through the ranks and built the respect and trust from all the individuals of the healthcare team. She was the driver of nursing excellence as the Chief Nursing Officer at a large hospital system in Michigan.

In 2013, about three years ago, she made the move to rural health with a drive to deliver the unexpected in healthcare. Kris leads a multidisciplinary team focused and dedicated on striving for the best. She has two Master's Degrees; a Master's Degree in Nursing and a Master's Degree in Health Administration. Great credentials! Great experience! I'm honored to have you here Kris, having this conversation.

Kris: Thank you, very much.

Bill: First of all, why did you choose healthcare as an occupation?

Kris: Well healthcare was second. I started out with business management and finance, which has really given me a great basis for healthcare, and then I was influenced by my mother who was a nurse.

After 15 years, I moved into healthcare and have never looked back.

Bill: Very interesting! There's so many of us that a great mentor had a big influence in our lives and our career. It sounds like that's what happened to you, for nursing specifically. There are many different ways you can get into healthcare. Was it primarily your mother's influence, or were there other reasons that you chose nursing?

Kris: My mom helped start me there, however, my ability to influence others and have an impact on someone's life has been something that I really liked once I started my nursing career. It drove through that focus of seeing how I could have the most time with my patients, and impact those patients. Just having that ability to have a positive impact on someone, to improve their life, was very influential.

Bill: That can be incredible, sometimes, can't it?

Kris: Yes, yes it can.

Bill: You have an interesting background because you were the Chief Nursing Officer at a large hospital system. Now, three years ago, you switched to rural health. Why the switch to rural health?

Kris: After working at the center and getting the experience, I moved through the ranks at the large system. I started out as a staff nurse, and worked up to charge nurse and manager, and then director, and then became the CNO. I did that quite quickly and for a variety of reasons. It gave me the opportunity to see where I could be an influence with rural health. Moving into a critical access hospital that was smaller, I felt that I could make a bigger difference quickly, as well as build a team that was instrumental to have the same vision. I felt that I could do that in a little bit better, more controllable manner, at a smaller facility as well as wearing a lot of hats, which is what I like. I still like to deliver patient care so I can throw on scrubs and take care of patients. It builds the ability to build respect with a team that says, "Hey, she'll walk a mile in our shoes."

Bill: Leading by example.

Kris: Yes.

Bill: In a rural hospital setting, you don't always have all the resources that you have in larger hospitals. Have there been any challenges for you in your transition to rural health?

Kris: It is definitely different. You hear a lot of different stories with regard to rural health whether you have the resources. I believe that when you have a strong team, you can look at every avenue that you need to, and build those resources from within, especially when you have a community that supports you. That's key for rural health. You build with the community around you, and then you have an army of more than just one. You can build off of those resources. It is a challenge, but again it's from building the team and some of those practices. Our hospital is independent. That's been one challenge because we want to remain independent as a critical access hospital. We have several large players that are big systems that we continue to work with and that is becoming more challenging. We are doing a good job with that, but it's been a challenge to stay independent.

Bill: I would think so, but it sounds like you're doing a great job there at Eaton Rapids Medical Center. I love talking about leadership, and I don't know if you watch the TV show American Pickers or not. Frank likes to collect oil cans and antique toys. I like to collect definitions of leadership. My next question is to add to that collection. What is your definition of leadership?

Kris: When I think of leadership, I think about collaboration. A collaborative leader that has the ability to influence others in not only direct reports, but all individuals, to influence them. A collaborative leader has the ability, to influence others through a very respectful relationship, all while holding them accountable.

Bill: I love that! Collaborative is a key word there. Influence is another key word you used, along with the ability to influence, which is vital to leadership. I like how you talked about that in a very respectful way. That's cool! With your permission, I'm definitely going to add that to my collection. Our mutual interest in leadership is actually how I met you. It was last year at a conference in Michigan where you did a presentation on leadership. It sounded like a very unique program that you put together at your facility. Can you talk about that?

Kris: Yes! Something that seems to be lacking in healthcare is customer service. I say that because when we go to a restaurant, we expect good customer service right? Otherwise we're not returning to the restaurant, or the food wasn't good. Hospital and healthcare in general is making a turn towards customer service and service excellence. We partnered with Capstone leadership solutions. They are a couple of excellent, influential nursing leaders that work for a small hospital here in Michigan. We partnered with them to start focusing on our customer service. That was three years ago, right when I came here. We picked one thing to focus on, and that was willingness to recommend. Through initiatives with Capstone and a focus on customer service, we developed tools to be able to deliver exceptional customer service. You would think it would come naturally, but it doesn't. When you come into a hospital, patients expect us to save their life, they really do. Now, we have to save their life with a smile. That is what I say.

Whether you're doing compressions in a code, you're doing lab work, or you're having a meeting providing education on diabetes or a new medication, we need to do it with a focus on customer service and compassion. That doesn't always come natural in healthcare, and we're starting to make that a priority. Not only because of reimbursement changes and things like that, but it is the right thing to do. It's bringing us full circle. The leadership tools we have developed for our leadership team has given them the knowledge, as well as our staff, the to understand those things that we can do. Whether you enter a room and ask, "is there anything else I can do for you?" Or preemptively not letting people hit their call lights by making sure that we're doing rounding. We are focused on rounding on patients and being more proactive instead of reactive. Those are all the tools that we've implemented and I am so excited to say that we've been number one in the state for patient satisfaction for almost two years, through our HCAP scores. That's number one in the state of Michigan out of 132 hospitals. We've been number one!

Bill: That's incredible.

Kris: It is! And I directly relate it to the team that we've built, the leadership tools that we've given them and focusing on willingness to recommend. We deliver the unexpected. Patients know we care, and it has accounted to our volumes, and our financial strength. We have physicians and surgeons that are seeking us out. It has been a win-win, and I directly relate it to that.

Bill: That is incredible, and that's an incredible accomplishment, to be number one in the entire state. Was the leadership training and the development that you did primarily focused toward your nursing staff, or was that across multiple areas in the hospital?

Kris: Great question! It was the whole hospital, from front line staff all the way across the continuum. I don't talk about up and down the organization, I talk about across because we're all equal. It's from housekeeping to nursing to physicians to external physicians that come here for our specialty clinic and their staff as well. We have employee driven committees, like best place to work. For example, we're trying to focus on being the best place to work for retention. To accomplish that, we created a 2-page document of behavior standards that we are very serious in upholding. That is for everybody. We focused on this idea quite a bit of time as well as the other tools we create. Rounding is a big one for us. We round on all patients. We round on all employees, routinely. Again, just building relationships, and building on those encounters that happen all the time.

Bill: Correct me if I'm wrong, as I recall from talking to you about this, don't you have a quarterly workshop or ongoing workshop with all your staff for leadership development type activities?

Kris: Yes, we do. We have a couple of different models. We have LDI's is what they're called, Leadership Development Institute. We have those quarterly for all of our leaders. We have either outside speakers come in, or we have internal ones who have gone to conferences and bring things back. They do presentations on that, so we're always developing our leaders through different things that are happening here. Over the last year and a half, we have created SDI's, which are Staff Development Institute, and that is where 100% of the employees in the hospital attend a three-hour staff development focused on things that they have given us feedback on that they want more education on. Those are quarterly as well.

Bill: That's great! I like your emphasis on leadership of course, and I also like that when you talk about customer service and willingness to recommend, yes, it is important today for reimbursement purposes, but I liked it when you said, it's also the right thing to do.

Kris: Absolutely.

Bill: Thank you, Kris! So far you have shared some great information with us.
You have some outstanding accomplishments. Obviously, you're focused on leadership, Kris, so what you would say your top leadership strength is?

Kris: I'd say my top leadership strength is integrity. I believe in not being afraid to make myself vulnerable. I wear my heart on my sleeve. I jump in when I need to, but I'm always respectful, and I hold people accountable, but I think my number one leadership strength is integrity. I've built a very strong relationship with my integrity in regards to relationships with physicians and all the staff in the hospital.

Bill: The way you described that, it sounds like this has been very intentional on your part.

Kris: Absolutely! You made the mention in regards to walking a mile in their shoes. I definitely do that. We are all here for the greater good of the patient, and you can't argue, when you put the patient in the center of every decision, you just can't argue what's right for him.

Bill: You know, you saying that integrity is your top leadership strength doesn't surprise me based on your definition of leadership. Thank you for sharing that.

Kris: You're welcome.

Bill: What are some of the challenges that you face, or that your hospital faces currently?

Kris: I would say some of the challenges would be insurance and legislation. Those are two things that we continue to be challenged with every day. Critical access hospital legislation continues to be a challenge, like whether they're going to change the mileage rules for the distance you can be from another hospital. Those are things that continue to be on our radar. Those are sometimes short-term, but more long-term goals challenges. Strategic planning needs to be fluid for rural health. That's something that we need to do differently, but is also a challenge in the sense of you can't just have a three or a five-year strategic plan and continue to move forward. You have to consistently be changing to keep up with the times for us to remain independent. What are the services that we need to increase? Swing bed program, behavioral health in psychiatry, some of those types of things. Those are challenges for us, just as they are for others. Physician recruitment and retention too. We've been thinking outside the box on that, but all these continue to be challenges.

Bill: When you say thinking outside the box, were you talking about physician recruitment specifically, or also the swing bed program?

Kris: Really both. Because swing bed program for rural hospitals is something that only about 90 critical access hospitals have swing beds. Swing beds were created to build inpatient volume, which is one of your highest revenue areas. We didn't have that before I came here. I started it, and we are just booming. We have five beds in our inpatient unit that are designated for swing bed, and we've been consistently full. We're doing different services because you have to compete with other long-term care facilities, so we have to think outside the box. Then there is behavioral health and psychiatry. We have created a structure where we're pulling licensed clinical social workers into planned visits with providers.

We have a rural health clinic where we look at the total picture. For example, if a patient comes in for diabetes, but you know that their behavior influences their diabetes, at the same time they have an appointment with the doctor, we provide a social worker to talk to them with regard to their behavior. This has a big impact for the patient in managing their chronic disease and it also benefits our hospital financially. We can bill separately for behavioral health and the social workers. That's something that we're really building on and is desperately needed. Of course, that's true nationally as psychiatry and behavioral health are sorely lacking. That's something that we've really been looking at.

Then there are physicians. For physician recruitment and retention, we're using mid-levels for inpatient care, with a team that includes our medical director through our rural health clinic. They are seeing patients in the rural health clinic, plus they are managing inpatient care, so there is a continuum of care. You can see the same doctor that admitted you to the hospital at the clinic. That has been a great success. Working with those individuals has provided great satisfaction along with training opportunities.

Bill: Are all the physicians employees?

Kris: We have two physicians who are employed. They are both medical directors who work with our rural health clinic and oversee our inpatient.

Bill: Thank you. Very interesting things that you're doing.

Kris you've been in rural health for three years, but you have a unique perspective with your experience. In your opinion, what do rural health leaders need to do differently?

Kris: It's delivering the unexpected and focusing on service areas. Community is one thing that rural health has to do differently because you need your community to back you and to support you. You need to focus on service areas and make sure that the community is making you their first choice for healthcare, not going outside of their hometown to receive services, for whatever reason it may be. There has been a misunderstanding that smaller hospitals do not deliver quality care, and that's simply not true. There's new evidence that shows that rural hospitals actually provide better care. We've met all of our core measures 100%, so your chances are much better by coming into our ER with a heart attack over a larger facility. If you think our numbers are lower,. then you may hesitate to come to our ER, yet, we have excellent success. We are hardwired with best practices. Again, this relates to how we impact our patient outcomes. Rural health really needs to focus on that and show that our quality exceeds or at least meets that, and we can deliver.

Bill: Speaking of the community, is Eden Rapids Medical Center one of the larger employees in town?

Kris: We are. We have a couple of manufacturing plants, magnesium plants that are here that have quite a large employee base as well, but we are one of the largest.

Bill: You can't lose sight of that. Like you said earlier, you need to make all of your decisions based around patient care. When you are one of the larger employers in town, that's another critical aspect of being there.

Kris: Yes. The outreach that we do for community health is significant. For example, we hold free health fairs and we go to the senior center every month and do a presentation based on a variety of different health care topics. Whether it's DNR, five wishes, education, vaccinations, Ebola training, Zika training, whatever, we're there in front of the community delivering that.

Bill: Very good. Community involvement is, for the most part, something everyone can do a better job of. I have one last question for you Kris. Actually, it's two questions in one. You can answer it either way you want. What excites you the most about the future, or what scares you the most about the future?

Kris: Okay. I'm going to go with the scary part first.

I think what scares me the most is what's uncontrollable. Legislative decisions and legislative changes feel like they are out of our reach. We are in an election year so that is no surprise. What's going to happen? Insurance changes and reimbursement are the things that all are very scary. That continues to be at our forefront and we try to impact those decisions as much as possible, but those are definitely scary.

The thing that excites me the most for us here at Eaton Rapids, is to continue to deliver the unexpected. It really is exciting to see this happen day in and day out and see our volumes continue to grow. It is great to know that we are doing the right thing and that we continue to rank number one in patient satisfaction, and continue to deliver excellent, quality care in our community. Just being part of this team is amazing.

Bill: It sounds like you've done an amazing job, Kris. An especially amazing job with integrity.

Kris: Thank you, thank you so very much.

Bill: Kris, I really appreciate you sharing your experience in rural health leadership. Thank you so much.

Dr. Steve Barnett

In this interview, I spoke with the President and CEO of McKenzie Health System, Dr. Steve Barnett. Our conversation included many important rural health and leadership topics. We discuss the importance of staying up to date and being current with healthcare changes and the need to interpret information to better improve your rural health community. We delve into Dr. Barnett's pioneering work as an Accountable Care Organization, as well as the struggles involved in recruiting specialty physicians for rural health. These, and many other important topics, are examined and discuss in the eighth episode of *Rural Health Leadership Radio™*.

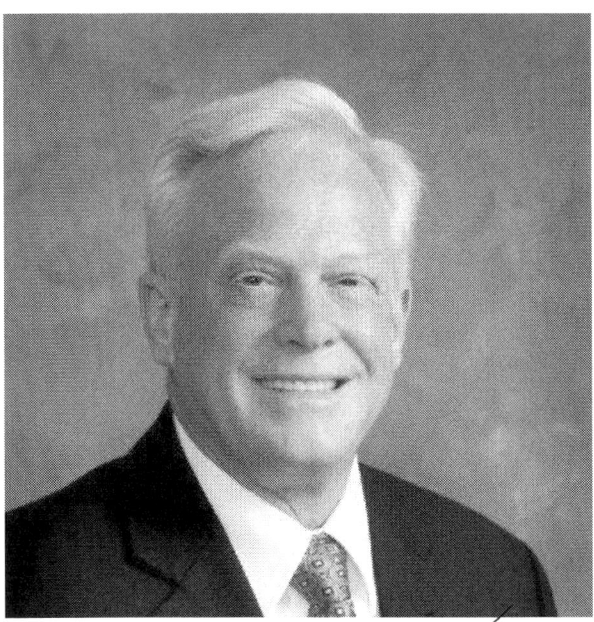

Bill: Dr. Steve Barnett has been the President and CEO at McKenzie Health System since 2008. During that time, Steve has provided leadership that has really shifted the culture of the organization, so much so that they now embrace change. McKenzie Health System is recognized in Michigan as a critical access hospital that is progressive and redesigning how healthcare can be delivered. Steve is a registered respiratory therapist, a registered nurse, a certified registered nurse anesthetist, and he has his doctorate in healthcare administration. A doctorate in healthcare administration, that's impressive, Steve. I'm shooting from the hip here, but I can't say that I know many CEOs at rural hospitals who have a doctorate in healthcare administration. Great credentials! Thank you for being on the show. Welcome!

Steve: Thank you! I appreciate it!

Bill: I want to get right into it Steve, to share what's working, what's not working, to share your experiences and your ideas and opinions on what's going on in rural healthcare. Before we really get into those questions, I'd like to ask you, why did you choose healthcare as an occupation path?

Steve: When I came out of high school, I didn't really have a good idea of where I was going to go or what I was going to do. I'm also one of the baby boomer people generationally, and I fell into it because I knew somebody who was a respiratory therapist. So, I ended up going in that direction. As you know, in Michigan, the automobile industry has always dominated the environment, so many people that I knew were going into that industry, most of them working on the line. That did not appeal to me at all, so healthcare is something that sounded like a good idea at the time, and, it's turned out that I've made a career out of it.

Bill: That's great. Did you have someone that mentored you in that process as you selected healthcare as an occupation?

Steve: Not really. I had a friend who worked as a respiratory therapist in one of the local hospitals in southeast Michigan. I was impressed with him and thought that might be something that I'd like to look into and explore further. I just fell into it really.

Bill: You had those influencing you, but you blazed your own trail it sounds like.

Steve: Pretty much.

Bill: Hey, whatever it takes to get there, right?

Steve: That's right.

Bill: Now the interesting thing is, you are from Michigan and you still live in Michigan. Michigan has a lot of large urban hospitals, but you chose rural. Why rural health?

Steve: I always wanted to work in a rural environment. When I grew up, where I grew up, although it's southeast Michigan, it was on the northern end of southeast Michigan, and at that time we were considered somewhat rural as compared to say, Detroit. I had worked as a respiratory therapist in a trauma center in Pontiac, Michigan, and then in surgical ICU in Detroit, Michigan. It's pretty exhausting. There are so many layers, and sometimes it's difficult to get things done. When I became a nurse anesthetist I really had a goal of moving into a rural environment that would afford me the ability to do a lot of things independently. This would open the door to provide a service that sometimes is difficult to find in rural environments. I finished that program off and came back to Michigan and ended up working in a multi-hospital system and very academic environment. It just took a little time, about 5 years, before I finally said, "Okay, it's time to pursue the rural piece." That's when I ended up in rural Michigan.

Bill: One of the things I always like to ask guests is, what is your definition of leadership? How would you define leadership, Steve?

Steve: I think you need to be current. You need to have a good idea of what's going on in your industry, and interpreting that information is quite often required because not everyone has the ability, or the time, that you need to really chew on some of the things that we have to read and try to translate into processes or things that we might do locally. That can all be overwhelming for many people, so you try to turn it into bite size pieces that everyone within the organization can grab hold of and accept. Then you start working on how others within the organization might adapt theses ideas to their environment. This process is really where I find a lot of my work lies. I feel that's a good deal of the leadership component. I think modeling the behavior that you're expecting from people obviously is critical, so blending those two things together is where I spend a lot of time.

Bill: I really appreciate the concept, the words you used were, "interpreting of the information." Interpreting information are the words that remain in my mind. I like that aspect of your definition. Thanks for sharing that. As a leader, as the President and CEO of McKenzie Health System, what would you say your top leadership strength is?

Steve: I tend to focus on our weaknesses rather than our strengths so it takes a little bit of thought for me to try and think of what that might look like. I really think it comes down to being believable. I say that because people aren't going to follow, they're not going to get behind the sort of activities and changes that you're often asking people to consider if what you're describing is not believable, and if you as an individual are not believable. I think being believable also leads to a level of trust and acceptability that people need for them to be willing to follow.

Our organization, like many small organizations, paint the walls or put pictures on the walls that represent the local geographic area. You ask people to go out and get some snapshots and then we frame them and hang them on walls. As you walk down the hall towards the med-surg unit, you can see them at our hospital. The director of nursing one day said, "Take a look at this, and walk with me." She walked me down the hall and pointed at this, that, and something else. They were all recognizable geographic areas in the local area. When we were at the end of the hallway, she asked, "What do you see?" I said, "I saw a lot of nice pictures." She said, "No, no, no, no, no." She said, "This is a journey. You're taking us on a journey. We're not sure where we're going, but we're okay with that. We're going to follow you."

Bill: That's great.

Steve: That was what she was trying to portray in the pictures.

Bill: What a great story. I do love it when hospitals do that. I always enjoy checking out what's hanging on the walls of a hospital. What a great metaphor that she led you down the hallway on that journey, because you're believable. It's interesting. As you said, that leads to trust. When you said believable the first thing that popped into my head was, "That's the way you create trust. When people believe you, you've created trust." That's certainly a strength! Thank you for sharing that.

Steve, I know you've done some interesting things at McKenzie, can you talk about something unique that you've done that's worked?

Steve: Since the Affordable Care Act passed in 2010, there was that initial push for the formation of Accountable Care Organizations. We heard a lot about Pioneer ACOs, but nothing had really been modeled, particularly for the rural environment. Regardless, we began to explore it further. We believed that it was obvious; focusing on how to keep people well is, in the long term, going to be far less expensive than what we've been doing for decades. It made a lot of sense to go down that path, the problem was finding an organization that we could work with, that could help us interpret claims data, because that's not an area that we typically had a lot of experience. That's really been the payer domain.

We took a couple of shots at trying to partner with organizations that were looking for lives, and those lives could be accumulated in rural environments. It never felt quite right, primarily because any of the funds associated with this endeavor were really going to be consumed by that claims data warehousing and analytics. There was nothing left over to really change how we were delivering care locally. Then I stumbled across an organization in 2013 called The National Rural Accountable Care Organization and became a founder of that entity. That's when we started putting together all the pieces and trying to make it work. We've been going pretty hard since; we're pretty excited about that.

Bill: You actually helped pioneer this effort, not just at McKenzie, but across the country?

Steve: Yes! While unique at the time, by now, most people listening, if they're in a rural environment, have probably heard of The National Rural Accountable Care Organization, and/or Lynn Barr. We organized 4 hospitals, critical access hospitals in northern California, a couple of hospitals in Indiana, and then us and an FQHC in Michigan. That became the founding group that we pulled ourselves together on lives and applied for application with CMS. We were approved as Medicare Shared Savings Program. That's where we started. That's how we began to identify what we need to make this work.

Bill: Great! A major accomplishment, not just for your facility but for others around the country. Thank you, Steve.

What a great success story about being an ACO and as one of the pioneers of ACOs in rural health. It sounds like that's something that you did that certainly worked, but quite often we learn a lot from things that we try that don't work or don't turn out the way we have planned. Can you share something that you tried that didn't work, or didn't turn out the way you'd planned?

Steve: Yeah, there are probably a number of examples.

The one that comes to mind, and we still struggle with this as do many of my peers, is recruiting specialists, and quite frankly, even recruiting primary care sometimes. What we try to do, or what always made sense to me is part of the problem. That is recruiting somebody to a rural environment who has a specialty and them not feeling as if they had fallen into the abyss because they have no collegial interaction or peer support. It's always a struggle when they want to take time off or get CEUs. Partnering with a larger organization is one way to solve this dilemma. Let's take cardiology for example. We recruited a cardiologist from a group from a larger nearby system to come here to see patients. It makes sense that traffic that needs to go to a larger organization would flow back to the entity they are affiliated with. This creates a win-win sort of relationship.

That's still been a struggle. It's hard to get some of these physicians to believe that there are real opportunities, and quite frankly, probably better opportunities in a rural environment than they might struggle with in an urban environment. That model has not worked out as well as I had hoped, but I think it's still a good one, and we'll keep hammering away at it.

Bill: Sure, good luck with that. Steve, you've had different roles, you've worked in urban centers, you worked in rural health What do you think rural health leaders need to do differently?

Steve: I think they really need to consider where we're going. They may not like it but they need to take a realistic examination of what's going on around them and find a way to begin to move their organization in that direction. What you don't want to do, or what I fear most, is that urban organizations are going to begin to acquire some of these rural facilities. What I expect would happen in that scenario, or I believe often does happen, is the urban facility is going to stamp that urban delivery system on that rural environment. Having been on both side of that fence it's not going to work; there are clearly some unique aspects. I hope that people begin to figure out how to drive that conversation and how to turn that around so that they don't end up losing that rural footprint, that presence.

Bill: Yeah, it would be a shame to lose it. What scares you the most about the future Steve?

Steve: Scares me?

Bill: Yes. Rural health as we all know, one in three rural hospitals have been identified as at risk, and they might close. We've had unprecedented closure rates of rural hospitals. It's a big thing. What scares you most about the future?

Steve: I think it is that closure, or that acquisition that I was just describing, where we lose the ability to still adapt care and how it's delivered to that local environment. The local being rural is much different than those urban environments. People are going to lose in that scenario.

Bill: That is scary. Let's flip that question around; what excites you the most about the future?

Steve: We're really at the forefront; primary care has finally risen to the level where it's going to drive everything. Rural environments really are a primary care specialty area. If you begin to think about it that way, and I would bet that 80% to 90% of what most people need to have done to them can be done within these rural environments, particularly with technology expanding the way it is. We're significantly reducing the amount of work that people historically have had to travel for. They do not need to do that anymore.

Bill: Having a rural hospital right where you are in rural America makes all the difference. If you can get things taken care of there, that makes a big difference. It may be the difference between life and death.

Steve: Absolutely.

Bill: One of the things that you've touched on a couple times now is not waiting around for an urban organization to acquire your facility. What have you done at McKenzie Health to prevent your facility from being acquired by an urban system?

Steve: It was in 2010, actually. We had been having a conversation, we being, myself and the board, about changing the relationship between another critical access hospital that's adjacent to ours. It's about 30 miles away. As is typical in most rural environments, everybody competes. Every town has its pride, and they want their own organization; they want to be able to do everything. Today we see it with municipalities; we see it with education; everybody is trying to find a way to consolidate and do a better job with fewer financial resources.

As they changed over their leadership, we took the opportunity to have a conversation to begin to looking forward. We asked, "How do we come together and quit beating each other up in an environment that is going to require we go the other way and work together and really manage our resources better?" That conversation took a few years, but in 2013 we were able to organize both these small hospitals under a new parent company. We continue to look for opportunities to not duplicate some of the managers or some of the services or some of the back-office stuff and recruit together. I think that puts us in a position where we're a little bit more offensive, where an urban or tertiary facility may look at us differently than if we were just standing here alone, and letting us kill each other. I think that was a good plan.

Bill: Interesting! A little bit of outside the box thinking in that. Earlier, you were talking about the pioneering work that you did to operationalize as an ACO. Is there anything else that you'd like to share about that?

Steve: Nothing other than it's a vehicle. Right now, the rules of the road and the opportunities are changing at a very, very fast pace. By the time this has aired who knows what we'll be dealing with, particularly in an election year. One thing that's probably not going to go away is a requirement to change how you deliver care so that the focus is less on sickness and more on wellness, and looking for programs and payers that want to embrace that and help you model how you change that care delivery so that you have adapted. It's not something that happens overnight; you've got to begin to understand it. You need to believe it. You need to find a good partner, which is what I was describing earlier. We partnered with the NRACO. Those folks, they're unique and they get it. Find the right partner and you will do well.

Bill: Great, thank you. I have one last question for you. You're a respiratory therapist; you're an RN; you're a CRNA; you have a doctorate in healthcare administration; most of those are clinical degrees, and you worked in those clinical settings for those respective degrees. How has your clinical background helped you as a hospital leader?

Steve: It has absolutely helped me! There are a number of conversations that we can imagine participating in, where you're working or working with a clinician or you're trying to recruit a clinician. The minute they discover that you have that clinical background, clearly a wall drops. Some of that, "Oh, you understand me," or, "You will understand my needs in the future." They're not asking necessarily that you give them all the toys that they're going to want or agree with all the recommendations they might make, but it changes the conversation and the tone of the conversation because they at least believe that you understand what their needs are. If you use that to work with them, it can be a really good relationship as you move forward.

Bill: You know what I enjoyed about the answer you just gave to that question Steve? It is the aspect that you talked about how they believe you. That goes back to what you said is your top leadership strength, that you are believable. Nice way to wrap up our conversation, by going back to that. Thank you, Steve, so much for sharing what you've done, what's worked for you, what hasn't worked and your other knowledge and experiences that you bring to the table from rural health to share with other rural health leaders.

Cody Mullen

In this episode of *Rural Health Leadership Radio™* we discuss rural health and leadership with doctoral candidate and Network Development Coordinator for the Indiana Rural Health Association, Cody Mullen. Cody shares success stories of rural health facilities in Indiana with regard to remote patient monitoring and health coaching programs. Cody also sheds light on the lack of legislature aimed specifically at rural healthcare. Together we expand upon many important topics in this interview.

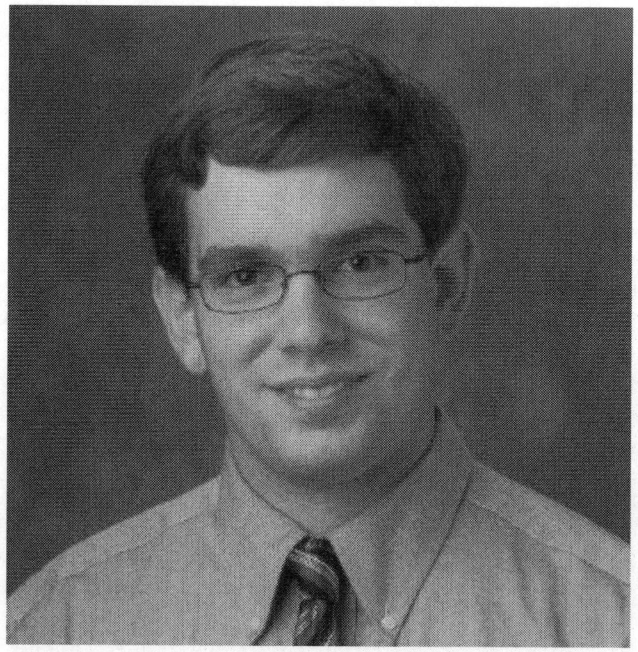

Bill: Cody Mullen is a doctoral candidate serving as the Network Development Coordinator for the Indiana Rural Health Association, what I like to refer to affectionately, as IRHA. Cody is, as the Network Development Coordinator for IRHA, facilitating the development of a remote patient monitoring and health coaching program to help lower the cost and improve the quality of care for individuals with a chronic disease or chronic condition. In addition, Cody supports the research and evaluation activities of IRHA.

He earned his bachelor's degree from Purdue University in Interdisciplinary Science, with a focus on healthcare engineering and statistics. He's currently a doctoral candidate in Health Policy and Management at the Richard M. Fairbanks School of Public Health, with a research interest in quality of care and access to care for vulnerable populations, especially citizens of Rural America and individuals with an intellectual or developmental disability. Cody is also an adjunct faculty member at Ivy Tech Community College in Lafayette, and is an associate instructor for the Fairbanks School of Public Health, where he's a doctoral candidate, at IUPUI, IUPUI being Indiana University-Purdue University Indianapolis. Cody's also a past NRHA Fellow. Cody! Great credentials! Welcome to *Rural Health Leadership Radio™*!

Cody: Thank you, and thanks for having me.

Bill: We met at the National Rural Health Association meeting. Actually, I sat in on your presentation first before we met, and I was very impressed with the work that you and IRHA are doing with chronic disease management. We'll get more into that in a minute, but first, I have a few questions for you. The first question is, what is your definition of leadership?

Cody: My definition of leadership would be an individual that has a vision that has been jointly developed by the people that they're leading, and helps support them in achieving that vision that they each have as an individual and as an organization, ensuring that everyone is having a part in fulfilling the vision of which everyone has set.

Bill: That is a very participative definition of leadership. I like the word "vision." Vision is always key to leadership, so thank you for sharing that definition.

Cody, you're working on your doctorate and you have a lot of academic credentials. You could have chosen a lot of different ways to go with your career. Why did you choose healthcare?

Cody: I like the word "vision." Vision is always key to leadership, so thank you for sharing that definition.

Cody, you're working on your doctorate and you have a lot of academic credentials. You could have chosen a lot of different ways to go with your career. Why did you choose healthcare?

Bill: That may be true, but the systems can drive you crazy, Cody.

Cody: True! There is never a dull moment, but if you, as my mentor taught me as an undergraduate, if you get those core skillsets under your belt, and if you get frustrated in one area to the point where you just want to scream and leave, you don't have to leave healthcare. You can transition from inpatient care, to outpatient care, urban to rural, or rural to urban. There're a thousand different ways that you can go with your work, but all that has a meaningful impact.

Bill: I believe you live in Lafayette, Indiana. Is that correct?

Cody: Correct.

Bill: Lafayette is more urban area, but you've chosen to work in rural health. Through the IRHA, you travel around the state to the rural hospitals and clinics. Why have you decided to focus on rural health? There are plenty of opportunities for urban healthcare centers in Indiana.

Cody: I list Lafayette as my ZIP code address, but I really live out in the country. I wake up every morning and look upon a field. I went to a county school, one of the biggest events that our school had was the, "Drive your tractor to school" day.

Bill: We had that too, where I grew up. We loved that day!

Cody: You know, I'm fortunate that within 5-10 minutes, I can be on one of the premier research universities campuses, top 100 universities in the country. And in five minutes, I can be standing in the middle of soybean and corn fields without seeing a soul. I can go to the county north of me, the high school is only in 20 minutes, and that's a county without a hospital. Where I live on this side of the county, we get healthcare in emergency situations. But for them, they have to drive a half hour to get to where I'm at, and then still drive another 20 minutes for healthcare. Realizing these differences in access to healthcare helped me see the need for rural healthcare and how it differed.

I also had a great mentor as an undergraduate. We were working on a project that was very urban-focused, working with a major health system out of Florida, and my mentor said, "What if we applied our approaches to a small, rural system?" We looked at 8 critical access hospitals and their hospital remission rates. I had no clue what a critical access hospital was before that point. With the system's approach, studying them, it was interesting to see their uniqueness and the difference they have.

Cody: This realization really excited me, but then, what really excited me was when you do a legislature research and query the legislature based on any topic that we were interested in, and add in the keyword of "rural." The number of articles that were produced in that search were next to none. It's a very underutilized research area. That showed me that there's a need and an opportunity to make a meaningful impact.

Bill: Interesting. It sounds like your mentor helped open your eyes to that.

Cody: Absolutely! He did a lot in the one year that we worked on that project that really changed the trajectory of my career.

Bill: The power of mentoring is amazing. It goes both ways for both the mentor and the mentee, another critical piece of leadership. When we talk about leadership, everyone has different strengths, skills, and opportunities for improvement. What would you say your top leadership strength is?

Cody: I'd say listening. I think a leader needs to do more listening than they do speaking. I've worked hard, through everything I've done, to try to be as thoughtful of a listener as possible, so when a decision needs to be made, if it can't be made collectively, all the facts are there so the leader is able to make a decisive decision.

Bill: I was always taught that you have two ears and one mouth, so you need to listen twice as much as you talk. Let's talk about what you're doing through the Indiana Rural Health Association with the chronic disease program that you have developed and created. Can you give an overview of what you're doing in that regard, Cody?

Cody: The Indiana Rural Health Association, or IRHA, is the home of the Indiana Statewide Rural Health Network, or InSRHN. This is the network that was formed with funding from the Federal Office of Rural Health Policy at the HRSA to become the stand-alone network to support our hospitals through shared learning collaboratives, shared contracts, and shared grants. We received funding, and we received a planning grant to plan that, and then a two-year funding opportunity to further develop that. Then it was off and running. We had 30 members when the next round of funding came out, so we went to our hospitals and asked, "We had this opportunity to go for this funding. We qualify based on the RFP's requirements. What would be the most helpful to you as you navigate the healthcare system?"

This was late-2013, early-2014 when this conversation was happening. The Affordable Care Act had just been passed; we were starting to become more knowledgeable of what all that entailed. Two of our hospital CEOs came to us and said, "We're joining the National Rural Accountable Care Organization," the NRACO. "We are transitioning to a value-based model. We have great clinical staff, but they're not training on how to do that long-term chronic disease management relationship so vitally important for an ACO to have. It would be great if we could have a real opportunity to train our staff, and get their skillsets in this area, better suited. It would also be of great value to get technology to help them do their job at a quicker and easier rate."

We wrote a grant and went to the HRSA again. Their response was, "What if we were able to train 10 coaches per facility in our network, as well as giving them a remote patient monitoring tool to support that?" HRSA was gracious enough to fund us, and we started our project in May of 2014. After we started the project, we quickly saw that the marketplace, and healthcare market, were totally changing. The ACO that started was just the first of those changes. A year later, the Chronic Care Management code came out. This is a code that if we provide 20 minutes of care coordination for a patient and we do a few other things, this is a billable service. In Indiana, it's billable at a rate of $38.88 per patient, per month, of utilizing that service.

This is an opportunity that you're going to get shared savings by doing care coordination properly. You're also going to start getting payment reports. You could support this division of your facility, either a clinic or a hospital, through this additional revenue. It's also helps the patient be more engaged in their healthcare, and makes sure their healthcare is at the utmost quality. Rural is already great at that, delivering quality healthcare, but ensuring that when they leave the rural market and go into the urban, first touch was with us, versus a different system. All that information is shared across the consumer care.

Bill: Very interesting. One of the things that you have done and you talked about briefly, is the idea of health coaches.

Bill: Can you talk about that? Who are these people? What kind of training do they have?

Cody: We have formed a strong partnership with the Iowa Chronic Care Consortium, or ICCC for short. They're based in Iowa, and they did a demonstration project several years ago looking at the Medicaid population of Iowa who have diabetes. They were able to show with their technique that they were able to bend the cost curve for that population in about two years. That really caught the eyes of my colleagues and our staff, as well as the hospitals that asked for this grant program. We went to them, and they said that they would come into our state to train our staff. Their training is an online curriculum, as well as a two-day intensive, where participants can practice the skills they've learned online. We really focus on three main areas.

One is motivational interviewing. How do you engage the patient in identifying where they'd like to make change? We seek understanding as the person helping them and why they want to make that change.

Secondly, we want to do goal-setting, and work on various goals. We focus on how do we do that, how do we develop smart goals, how do we engage the patient on their own goals that they've developed, and then how to achieve them.

Thirdly, how does the personality type of that patient differ with how we do coaching? If I had a very introverted thinker, I'd change my approach than if I had an extroverted feeler, for example.

How, as a coach, can I quickly pick up on cues from my patients, to know the personality type? Then we train with, "Okay, if they're that personality type, that means this will affect them differently, so I should frame it as this type of problem, or this type of question, versus that." All that is incorporated in our curriculum. We have now trained over 120 coaches around Indiana. We support them and help them feel comfortable going out and doing this, developing a long-term relationship with their patients.

Bill: What kind of background do those coaches have prior to the coach's training? Did they come from a variety of backgrounds?

Cody: They all have a very broad background. The training is an add-on skill, so the patient comes in and says, "I'm really struggling with how this medication makes me feel." The coach is going to rely on training that they've already had to build a system with that information.

We train a lot of LPNs and RNs through this program. They're probably our most common background, but we've trained everything from a personal trainer at the YMCA, a church member who's starting a church group; we've trained hospital CEOs; nurse practitioners, paramedics, exercise physiologists and pharmacists. It's very broad on who goes through the training. The training really meets them where they're at and helps them move forward in their own skill and personal development. We find that the best model is when we can train a diverse group of individuals throughout a system.

We can train a base of nurses, five or six nurses, that are going to do a lot of the coaching as part of their job. We can also train an exercise physiologist, a pharmacist, and a nutritionist. If that patient has really unique or detailed concerns, questions, or assistant needs, they can refer them back up to someone who has a higher clinical training in that area. The patient really is feeling the same approach as their normal coach, but has a higher, more unique skillset in answer to the unique questions that they have.

Bill: Very interesting! Cody, thank you for sharing that information about this program. It's been in existence for a little over 2 years now. What has been the biggest, or perhaps, the most significant impact this program has had to date?

Cody: You know, we are still evaluating. I can share some of the anecdotal impacts that we have felt. These aren't coming from an evaluation report but we're seeing huge effects on patients. Patients are more engaged in their healthcare than they've ever been. Patients are enjoying having someone that they can talk to on a monthly basis about their healthcare concerns. Patients don't have to wait until they see the doctor, or don't feel bad because they feel like they can't ask the doctor simple questions because they're on such a tight timetable. We're hearing great patient engagement stories, patient activation stories, near-misses or near-catastrophes for patients.

Through the monitoring system, the coach has been able to engage with patients before it becomes an adverse event, and the patient didn't know that they were nearing an adverse event, the health coaches have been able to engage them, which has had a huge quality of life improvement for the patient, as well as savings for the facility.

We're also hearing facilities tell us that this is empowering them in the value-based transformation that these facilities, that all of our healthcare system, is moving towards.

This process is engaging their staff and getting them ready for a full-on capitation payment model that may be coming down the pike, and it's helping them feel better when seeing massive releases of different models. They can say, "Oh, this is how coaching fits with that. We're always doing part of this, and all we've got to do is add this, or this, or this," and they will be ready.

Bill: Interesting! Anytime you implement a new program like this, it doesn't always go as smoothly as you'd hoped. When implementing change, it's inevitable that you may have to be flexible during implementation. What aspects of this program weren't going the way you had planned on, that you had to make some modifications or some tweaks along the way?

Cody: We've really changed, over the three years we've been doing this. Our approach and our "sales pitch" to our patients and the hospitals we're working with along with the staff within those hospitals. When we first started this program a little over two years ago, the terms, "population health" and "value based payment models" were not as readily known as they are today. We've gone from educating on, "What is population health?" to "How does this fit into population health?" That's been a big change there. We've also changed our education approach to our patients and our clinicians.

Bill: Some clinicians feel very guarded, that the coach is coming in to take over their patient. They feel like it means they are not doing their job right, and that's why the coach is coming in. We've really worked on developing ways as to how the practice is implementing this, to see how this fits within the overall picture of healthcare and consumer of care, that this is a piece that's not replacing anything, it's really just an added piece to help tie it all together.

Cody: I'm guessing that the concept of the health coach was a new concept when you implemented this? You know, two years ago, it was a very new concept. A lot of people weren't sure how that fit in. Now, a lot of people have heard about it, and they're coming to us, saying, "Hey, I hear you're doing health coach training. What kind of health coach training do you do, and how do we get involved?" I mean, that's a shift of the times as well.

Bill: Yes, and change, can be scary. I can understand the second-guessing. "Why do you need a coach? I'm taking care of the patient." That's a change that had to be implemented there. It sounds fascinating; I'm very intrigued by this. Not every hospital CEO, not every state hospital association has the structure that allowed you to put this program together. From what you've seen, what can rural healthcare leaders in other areas of the country learn from what you're doing in Indiana?

Cody: We're more than happy to talk to anyone, and share in a lot more detail about what we did, and how we did it. Some of the partners that we brought to the table, because some of those partners could also be brought to the table in other states. Our training partner and technology partner had never met before, but we pulled them together and said, "Here's what we're doing." They've worked and developed things in tandem.

That helps, but it's really just start small. When we started this, we trained 20 coaches and engaged about 100 patients. That was it. Now we're engaging over 1000 patients, and have over 100 coaches, and it's taken 2 years, so it's not an area that we throw on the light switch and automatically, we have a coaching department. There is an education period; there is a comfort period that takes time to build into this program.

Bill: It sounds like the patients like the health coach. Is that your perception?

Cody: Yeah, our perception is that patients really enjoy this, and that's what literature has shown over the life of studying those areas and the patient. It wasn't for the first time, but a lot of patients enjoy talking with clinicians, and enjoyed having that support system. Knowing that, "In a week, I can ask these questions, I don't have to save that up." This is an avenue, an opportunity that we give them to be able to ask those questions, be able to give them that framework, and be able to help them achieve the goals that they may have had for themselves for a very long time, to start achieving them.

Bill: Great! As you can tell, I'm fascinated with this idea. That's very generous for you to make yourself available to talk to other health, rural health leaders in other parts of the country on your experiences. You've seen a lot of different rural hospitals; you've implemented this new program. Is there anything that you would like to see rural health leaders doing differently?

Cody: I don't know if it's differently, because, you know, I'm young in the field; I'm still in school. I don't want to sound like I'm making recommendations and not knowing the historical reason for why we are where we are, but I think embracing value-based care, accepting that, and knowing that its forthcoming, and not being fearful of it is something rural health leaders may want to do differently. It's there to improve clinicians; it's there to improve patients. It will even improve our country. Just being able to embrace that, and understand that it is hard, it is confusing, it is going to take some time to get used to it. But once you do, you won't want to turn back.

Bill: Well, don't apologize for your newness in the industry, Cody, because we always need fresh eyes looking at what we're doing. I appreciate your perspective very much.

As I’m sure you know, one in three rural hospitals have been identified as "at risk” of closing, so this is serious stuff we're talking about. You've mentioned that where you live, people in the next county have a far way to go to get to a rural hospital, or any hospital for that matter, and that could be very scary. What scares you most about the future?

Cody: I think what scares me most is that decisions about healthcare are going to be made about the areas where the biggest expenditures are, which is the urban tertiary advanced care centers. Then, the cost here, those would be the rural providers that ride the basic life-sustaining care that's needed for a healthy country. It's very simple to say, you know, "This makes up 20% of the overall budget, so let's focus on the 80% area that they cost, and not worry about the 20% area," but that 20% area is not providing the optional services, or the services that people can travel to. That's the people that are five minutes down the road for a heart attack at 2:00 am, or full labor and delivery, and the lady is in a breach position, needs immediate supports to save both mommy and baby. These rural providers need to be able to stay and do their job, and not be worrying about, "Are the lights going to be turned off tomorrow?"

Bill: Thank you for that perspective. Now, let me flip that question. What excites you the most about the future, Cody?

Cody: What excites me the most is that rural has always had the history of being the innovators of healthcare for the country. They're the first ones, they do it, and that's just the rural perspective. We do what we do, next to none, and we do it at the most cost-effective rate that we can do it at. That excites me. I'm excited anytime I go to a national meeting with the Rural Health Association, or any of the other associations that I visit with, to have that rural discussion with like-minded people. When I meet people who don't know rural and explain what we're doing; their eyes get wide and they say, "Wow! You guys are doing what we're hoping to be doing in 10 years."

Cody: We're already doing that in rural, and what we're doing is impacting the people that we know. In the urban market, I might never see my patients outside the hospital. In the rural market, they're at the basketball game on Friday night with you; they're at the football game; they're at the movie theaters; they're at 4-H. You know them; you see them; they're your community members. What we're doing is making their quality of life that much better.

Bill: Incredible. Thank you, Cody. Thanks for sharing what you're doing in Indiana, and what an incredible story. I love the chronic care program that you're facilitating there.

LIZ MONK

Bill: I sat down with Liz Monk, Director of Care Coordination at Munson Healthcare Grayling Hospital, for a discussion of rural healthcare and leadership in the following interview. We delved into many topics, such as the need for rural health facilities to be forward thinking to stay afloat, but the crux of the interview follows the ups and downs of Ms. Monk's work creating the hospital's collaborative partnership with rural health clinics, Joy in the Journey.

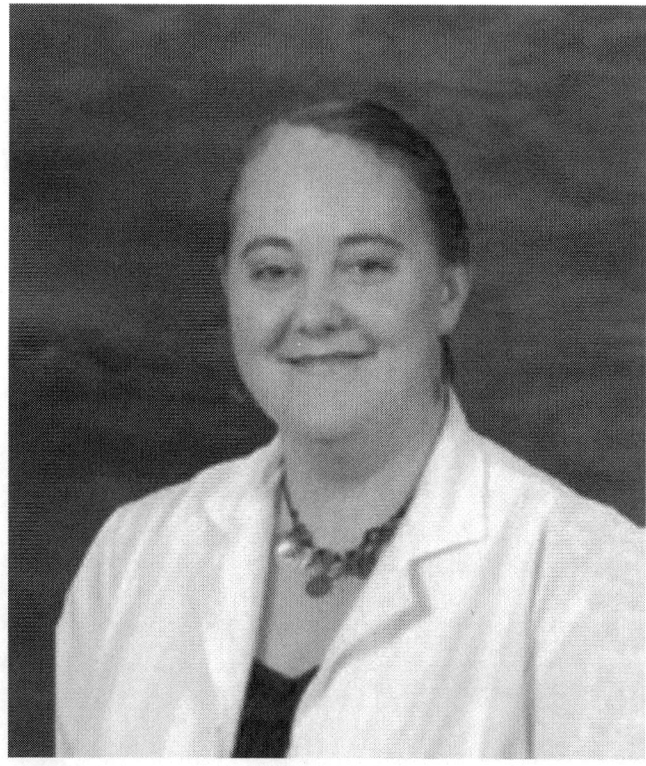

Bill: Today we're having a conversation with Liz Monk, the Director of Care Coordination at Munson Healthcare Grayling Hospital in Grayling, Michigan, which is part of a small health system consisting of a seventy-one bed community hospital, a long-term care facility, and three rural health clinics that serve a five-county area in Northern Lower Peninsula in Michigan.

After obtaining her Bachelor of Science in Nursing from Michigan State University, Liz gained clinical experience in the emergency department, in case management and physician performance and improvement. Her experience includes readmissions, performance improvement, and innovation. Prior to her nursing career, Liz's Bachelor Degree in Physiology led her to military service as an aero-medical technician at Davis-Monthan Air Force Base in Arizona, followed by her next role as an aero-space physiology officer at Moody Air Force Base in Georgia.

Liz, thank you for your service to our country, and thank you for your service to rural health, and most of all, welcome!

Liz: Thank you, Bill!

Bill: Let's get rolling, Liz! We want to share your knowledge, but the first question I want to ask you is why did you choose healthcare as an occupation? There're so many different career paths that we can choose these days, why healthcare?

Liz: I've always had a passion for helping people, which is kind of the stock answer, but the reason I went into nursing is because it gives me so many opportunities to really explore different areas. I've met some amazing nurses throughout my career path, especially in the military, that were doing such varied things, not just the normal, traditional bed-side nursing. They were able to get out and run practices and run projects and run operations. That's really what intrigued me about the nursing field and why I decided to go into that.

Bill: Did you have a particular person that mentored you in that process, that made a difference for you?

Liz: I've had a lot of mentors along the way, but I have to say, the first nurse that really mentored me was actually a school nurse that was teaching our healthcare occupations program in high school. Her name was Juanita Walt, and she lives in our area. She's just an amazing woman.

Bill: That's great. Mentors make such a difference in so many ways. Munson Healthcare Grayling Hospital is part of a larger health system. Where you are is more rural. Why did you choose rural health in your healthcare career?

Liz: Well, there're a couple of reasons. First, it's the community. When you get into a rural community, it's pretty spread out and you have to know your resources. Part of that is really creating strong partnerships with community members and other service agencies. I like that aspect of it, because I think as a community we can do much greater than we can individually. Even though rural is less focused, and has less resources, we really try to work as a bigger team to accomplish what we want to accomplish.

Bill: Did you grow up in the Grayling area?

Liz: I grew up near the Grayling area. After I left the military and decided to come closer to home, I actually looked at several of the hospitals in Northeast Michigan, and I chose Grayling because it has a phenomenal, quality program. They seemed to be at the time, and I know this is true now, really progressive in their thinking and very forward thinking. That's the type of hospital that I wanted to be in.

Bill: That's great! One of the questions I ask every guest is, what is your definition of leadership?

Liz: My definition of leadership is a little different than most. I tend to look at leadership as empowering the people that we lead to transform healthcare, through things like collaboration and innovation. I want to inspire people that I work for to move forward and to really look at evolving to a new way of thinking.

Bill: Does your military experience influence your definition of leadership?

Liz: I think it does. I was in the Air Force, and I was a specialist in human factors and human things that go into flying. Part of what I did was looking at aircraft accidents and stuff like that. I think with the way healthcare is going and really trying to follow in line with high reliability and transformation, I think that really influenced me in how we look at becoming better. It did influence it, and of course, the military is all full of leadership type courses, they're big on that, so I attended and took advantage of that. It caused me to think about how I wanted to be, as a leader.

Bill: I appreciate that very much. Part of my rationale for asking that question is that I was just reading a book written by a gentleman who was former military. He retired from the military and was talking about how some people challenge him on the fact that, "How can you use what you learned about leadership in the military in other applications, be it healthcare or any other industry?" He made a very powerful argument about how it's very true that you can do that, and the lessons that you learn in leadership in the military are applicable in so many different ways in all walks of life.

I really love the word you used in your definition about empowering people. You also used the words collaboration, innovation, inspiration, all great and powerful words that really make a great definition of leadership. Thank you for sharing that with us.

Liz: You're welcome.

Bill: For you, as a leader, you have military experience, you have clinical experience, you are now in a very important leadership role at your facility. What would you say is your top leadership strength?

Liz: My top leadership strength is really creating a vision and getting the people onboard to work towards that vision together. That's what we've been doing for the last few years. That's what we're going to continue to do as we move forward into the future, because with the changes that are occurring in healthcare, I think everybody who's in the overall community knows it's extremely important to be sustainable. For our rural hospitals to be sustainable, because I have patients that if we weren't here, they would have to travel upwards of an hour to get to the next nearest facility. To get them good healthcare, where it needs to be, we have to be forward thinking.

When you look at how we apply leadership principles in the rural community, we need to be ahead of the game. We need to be forward thinkers. We need to look at where things are going and be ahead of it, because we can't sustain the huge hits that some of the changes in healthcare have brought on. We had a hospital that was similar in size and nature to us in Massachusetts, and I kind of considered it a sister hospital when I was really working on readmissions work. They weren't doing great in quality. They weren't doing well on readmissions either, and within a year of the first penalty for readmissions, they closed their doors. We have to be ahead of that. We can't sustain those type of hits.

Bill: When it takes an hour to get to the closest hospital, that's a life and death scenario there.

Thank you for sharing that. You talk about creating a vision and getting people on board, and being forward thinkers. In a prior conversation that you and I had, you actually demonstrated how that is exactly who you are. You put together a very unique program to coordinate care between some rural health clinics and your hospital. Can you talk about that?

Liz: Sure. One of the goals that we wanted to achieve was based on stories we kept hearing about patients falling through the cracks. You hear about a patient that leaves your hospital and is supposed to go to the clinic, and nothing was set up right. Nothing was followed through. We just missed the mark. We really wanted to set up a system that helped to capture that, helped to ensure that there were smooth hand offs going on, that we had transitions, that we have better management of our patients that were really at risk for coming in the hospital and spending a lot of healthcare resources on them.

What I was charged with was creating an infrastructure for our system, to provide better care coordination across the system. Now, we've been about two years into this, and we still have a long way to go. We've only been focusing on certain segments of the population, some really vulnerable ones, and the work we're doing is laying the foundation for where we're going to be going to in the future. Essentially, what I've done is I've created a collaborative partnership with our rural health clinics in order to provide better care across the continuum for our patients.

Bill: There're three of those clinics, correct?

Liz: Correct. Those clinics are owned by our hospital, so they're employed. The three clinics, prior to my starting my work, were very segregated. It was the clinics and the hospital, and they were very separate entities. One of my biggest goals was to help break down those silos and bring everybody together to work towards the same purpose.

Bill: On a scale of one to ten, how challenging has this been? Has it been a ten or less than that? It sounds like a very intimidating task.

Liz: That's kind of my personality. You give me the hardest task, and that's what I like to do. That's where I like to spend my time. To me, it hasn't really been too bad. Three to four? There's times when it's jumped up a little bit more. Quite frankly, we had the right things in place. We had the right leadership. At the time that I was brought on to do this, they brought on a new director of practice operations that was very much on board with the vision. The senior leadership was one hundred percent behind this. This was their vision as well, so as we all came together and developed this. It was a very collaborative effort. Having the right partners makes it a lot easier task.

Bill: Absolutely, no doubt about that. I'm sure part of that was because of your leadership and the leadership of others to make sure that you could achieve that alignment. Thank you, Liz, for sharing that information about that program.

While you were implementing this program, Liz, were there any aspects of this that weren't necessarily working? If so, what did you do?

Liz: I think there are always challenges. We have a ton of aspects of our process that get broken all the time. I think constantly improving processes and adhering to the improvement cycle, really looking at process improvement all along really helps. That's exactly what we did. I've had instances where we were trying to figure out reporting relationships so that we could really get things moving in the right direction. Actually, we're still working on that. We've had instances where we had people reporting to me, that maybe it didn't really make sense. We had an OB Care Coordinator that was reporting to me, and it wasn't really working out the best because she needed more support on the OB knowledge and getting integration. She worked in the rural health clinics, but she really needed processes. The challenge with her was she was not integrating into the hospital side as well. We changed that to report directly to the manager of the OB department in the hospital, and that helped tremendously.

How we worked through that process, it was again, sitting the people down, the stakeholders down in the room and collaborating. The director of practice operations, myself, and the OB manager sat down and just talked it through. What makes sense with this? That adaptability and the flexibility within the program is what's really made it successful. We have some people on the operational side. Some of the practice operations people report directly to me, and some report to the offices or the functional service line. It really depends on where they need the most support. Having the understanding between myself and Mike Johnson, who is the practice operations director is key. We just sit down and hammer things out. We have this understanding between us and we do it in a very professional manner. Sometimes we step on each other's toes. Sometimes we'll say one thing, and I'll say one thing, and he'll say something else, but at the end of the day, we just come together and come to an agreement. It works out really well.

Bill: Sometimes it's more difficult to talk about than others when you have so many different groups that you're trying to coordinate. Sometimes there is a tendency for people to protect their turf. Have you had to deal with that? If so, how did you break down those barriers?

Liz: Yes, we have. As Mike will tell you, I steal all of his space. In order to implement these programs and get really good care coordination, one of the goals was to get chronic disease care managers in the offices. Those are my reports. I work on the hospital side, for the most part, so that's where my budgets are. We can't build. We don't have the extra operating income to be able to build new offices, so we have to make do with what we have. Sometimes that means fitting them into spaces. We've had a lot of turf wars, actually, where it's like, "I need space to do this work, Mike, what do you want me to do?" We just keep going back and forth until we figure it out. We brainstorm and bring in the managers of the different offices and say, "Okay, how can we do this?" It takes flexibility.

Because we don't have the space, one of my people right now is in the manager's office. The office manager leaves when she has a patient come in. It's that idea that we're all working towards the same goal, and we just need to do what we need to do to figure it out. Bringing people together and being flexible is a challenge, but we just keep working through it. Open communication is always the key.

Bill: Doing what's right for the patient I would think is probably overpowering.

Liz: Actually, we have this saying we use all the time. Our entire program is called “Joy In The Journey,” and it's bringing joy to the patient who's in the center of all we do.

Bill: Joy In The Journey?

Liz: Yes, it's Joy In The Journey.

Bill: I love that! You're in a unique situation here, implementing this program. What can other rural healthcare leaders take away from what you've accomplished?

Liz: I think the biggest thing is that we all need to start thinking differently. We need to look at collaboration and cooperation as the key to the future, rather than your own personal gain. You have to look at the bigger gain for the patient and the organization. It can be done quite successfully, if you're willing to step outside of your normal roles and responsibilities. You don't say, "That's not my job." You say, "How can we get this done together?" I think that's our biggest takeaway here. We've been thinking a lot differently as a system towards systems and cooperation.

The biggest challenge is, and what I think most people will find the biggest barrier implementing something like this, is saying, "Well, that's fine, but we don't own the practices, so we can't implement that." That's absolutely not true. One of the things I didn't want to lose sight of is we have other practices in the area, and we want to include them as we can. If they have the resources to really help integrate some of this work, then we bring them on board. We have collaborative meetings with care managers from other offices that look at some of their high-risk patients, and we collaborate back and forth on this type of stuff. We have a transitional care manager that works out of the hospital and serves all patients that are at high risk, not just the ones that we own.

Bill: Interesting. In integrating the non-hospital owned clinics, how does that transition compare to the clinics that are owned by the hospital?

Liz: It's definitely more challenging. Some come on board quicker than others. We had one practice that came on board and we reach out to them more. We had another one that was really engaged and doing quite well. Unfortunately, that practice closed recently. After they closed, a couple of the providers came to work for us, so I think it helped to build those relationships within the community. Historically, this practice hadn't had the best relationship with the hospital. It's a very different story today because of the collaboration that we started.

Bill: Great! You've been at this initiative for two years now. If you had to start it all over again today, what would you do differently?

Liz: I don't really know, because I think about some of the missteps that I took in the beginning, but I think they lent to some very valuable learning experiences. I don't know that there's much I would do differently, other than try to gain more experiences. We've implemented it, we've shown successful revenue generation and we have a much better experience for our patients.

I had to laugh the other day when one of my ER case managers came to me and said, "Let me tell you this story. I had a patient show up in the ER, and they were like, 'Well, wait a second, I've got to call my person, because before I talk to you, I need to call my person.' So she got on the phone and called one of our care managers in the offices." Well, I've integrated all of those departments, so when she called the care manager in the office, my ER case manager said, "Let me talk to her." She gets on the phone and she says, "Hey, how are you doing today?" They're talking back and forth, but she got a great report on what was going on with the patient. It's that type of interaction that we're seeing on a daily basis that
we've been able to accomplish. There was an ER case manager here a few years back, and today we're able to accomplish in two days what used to take a month and a half to do to coordinate care.

Bill: That's tremendous. Congratulations on your success, and continued success as you continue to implement this program.

Liz: Thank you.

Bill: Liz, with your experience in rural health and healthcare in general, what do you think rural health leaders need to do differently? You've kind of spoke to this already, but I'll go ahead and ask you that question anyway.

Liz: I think we need to collaborate. We need to collaborate locally with other providers, with other community agencies. As you said in the beginning, we're a small hospital in a larger system, and part of what I found is collaborating with our larger system gives us some benefits, too. The more we look into the future, and that patient that maybe would have to drive a hundred miles to get to the doctor, if I can think differently about how we deliver care, if I can bring some of the things that you have to go to the big city to get, to my hospital, to provide it more locally, how do we do that? Some of those answers lie with visiting specialists, sometimes that may lie with telemedicine, sometimes it may lie with something totally different. As leaders, we need to ask, "How do we do this differently, and how can we make this work?" If we don’t ask these questions, we're doing a disservice to our community, and we're not truly benefiting our rural community.

Bill: As we know, rural health has a lot of challenges right now. You've spoke to that in some of your comments here. What scares you the most about the future of rural health?

Liz: To be honest, what scares me the most is some of the systems that have been set in place won't allow us to think differently about how we need to deliver care in the future. I'll give you an exact example. Medicare wants providers to start providing an adult wellness visit. It's essentially a way to get through an assessment of a patient that's like a psychological, social, and functional assessment. It is a great assessment. You're not going to pay a doctor to do it because it takes an hour to an hour and half to accomplish. However, Medicare thought, "You know what? We see this as a problem, so we're going to let RNs do this." Because we are in a rural health area, and we get RHC reimbursement, that RN, under the RHC rules, can't do that without having a physician face-to-face. That has to do with the RHC billing rules. Some of those regulations hold us back with what we want to try to get accomplished.

We've been able to do it here. That's one of those things that you keep doing things differently until you figure it out. Essentially, we do have a nurse doing it, and then we have the physician coming in towards the end of it to look over the prevention plan. The whole point is to come up with a prevention plan for the patient, to keep them healthier. We keep running into restrictions like that, because some of the reimbursement things don't catch up as quickly with the way the government wants us to change to more quality and preventative type things like that.

Bill: Thank you for sharing your thoughts on that. Let's close with one last question. What excites you the most about the future?

Liz: The care we get to deliver to the patients. I think we're really thinking about some new and innovative ways to truly put the patient at the center, and that excites me. It excites me a lot.

Bill: That's the best part of all, isn't it?

Liz: It is! It is!

Bill: Thank you, Liz, for sharing your insights, your experiences in rural health along with some unique things that you have done.

Ryan Kelly

In this episode of *Rural Health Leadership Radio™*, the conversation is with Ryan Kelly, Executive Director of the Mississippi Rural Health Association. We cover a vast array of topics in a short span of time from the importance of cost reports in the survival of rural hospitals, and how there's more to the story, to the importance of making a rural hospital more than a hospital. Kelly helped create the Mississippi Rural Health Fellow program, a great resource for rural health leaders which is expanded upon in the following interview along with many other important and interesting rural health and leadership topics.

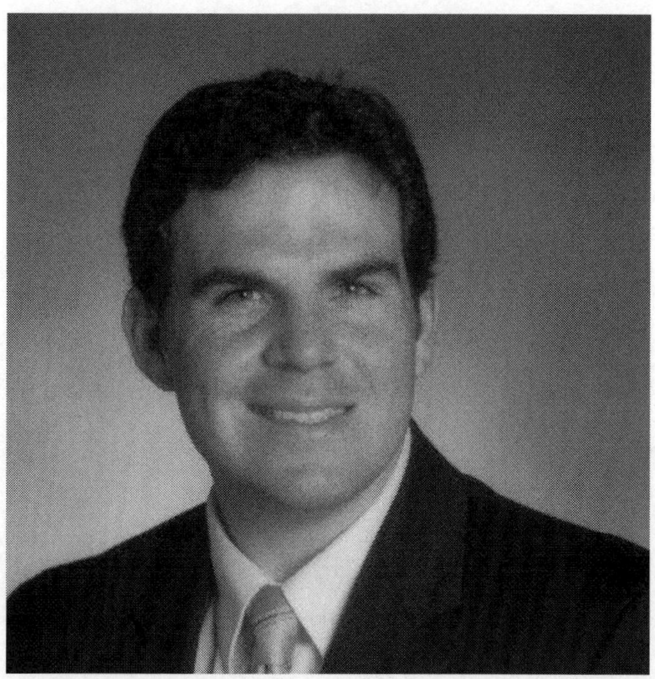

Bill: Today we're talking with Ryan Kelly, Executive Director of the Mississippi Rural Health Association (MRHA). Ryan is a Mississippi native. Prior to his leadership role at MRHA, Ryan served as the Chief Advancement Officer for William Carey University and Director of External Relations for the University of Southern Mississippi College of Health. Ryan earned a Bachelor of Science with Honors from the University of Southern Mississippi in 2005 and a Master of Science with Honors from Mississippi College in 2007. He's a member of the Area Development Partnership's Leadership Pine Belt, the Mississippi Economic Council's Blueprint Mississippi Committee, the Association of Fundraising Professionals, and the Mississippi Society of Association Executives.

In addition to professional activities, Ryan also serves as a Deacon at the Temple Baptist Church, an Advisory Board Member of the Children's Center for Communication and Development, and the United Way of Southeast Mississippi, the Gideon's International, Pi Kappa Phi Alumni Association, and most recently, as Chair of the Southern Miss College of Health Dean's Council. He's also served as the Chair of the Mississippi Health Summit over the past four years.

Bill: Ryan, you are a busy guy! Welcome!

Ryan: It's a pleasure to be here, Bill. Thank you.

Bill: Thank you! Let's jump right into the questions. Why did you choose healthcare as an occupation?

Ryan: The Lord opens up great opportunities for us throughout life, and healthcare was always one of these areas that I have had a passion for. Through a roundabout way of going through a university system, I ended up in health disciplines, working with a variety of healthcare professionals. I had the opportunity to start running this association and it has grown substantially over the years. I was able to fulfill what I always felt was a mission of mine, and that's being in and around healthcare. I enjoy what our physicians and our nurses do and I have great appreciation for all of our hospital and clinic administrators, our insurers, and just everyone who's involved in healthcare right now. Everyone has a part to play, and hopefully I'm filling at least one small role here in Mississippi, helping to advance healthcare forward.

Bill: That's great Ryan! I'm sure there're a lot of people that appreciate the contributions that you're making. Why did you choose to focus on rural health?

Ryan: I grew up right outside of Jackson, Mississippi, which would not be considered rural, but I've always had this rural heart. My family comes from rural Texas and rural Mississippi. They have lived and breathed tractors and growing crops and just everything about my family has been rural. I don't know whether it's genetic or environmental or what, but even though I've grown up in a semi-urban environment, I've always had this rural desire. I'm trying to convince my family to move back to the country.

Where we live now is more of a suburb of a slightly urban area. It would be great to have cows and chickens and all of the good things you think of when you think of rural Mississippi. I'm trying to work my way out that way. The people in rural are genuine. They're sincere. Not that anyone in our state is not, but it's just that the good things about Mississippi always typically fall with rural Mississippi. It's where my heart has grown and continues to grow every year.

Bill: It sounds like it might be part of your DNA, Ryan.

Ryan: Maybe so.

Bill: One question I always ask is what is your definition of leadership?

Ryan: That's an excellent question. You can read all sorts of books from John C. Maxwell or other leadership executive. I love reading those because everyone's perception is just a little bit different, but leadership is definitely not a job title. It's not getting a promotion into an area. It's not how much money you make or don't make. Leadership is, in my opinion, the perception that others have of you. As an example, there were two nuns that were recently unfortunately tragically murdered here in Mississippi. They had nothing. They were nurse practitioners in a clinic. They were seen as leaders in that community.

Leaders do not have to have high salaries or big titles. They have to be respected by others. They have to form a bond with those around them, and others have to trust them and lean on them and depend on them. When I think of leaders in our state, I don't necessarily think of those in elected positions or those that are the head of big companies. I think of those that others look up to, those that others depend on. And that, for me at least, is leadership.

Bill: Thank you, Ryan. I appreciate you sharing that. That certainly was tragic news about the nuns who were killed. I do appreciate that you include in your definition or your description of your definition that you don't have to have a title to be a leader or you don't have to be promoted to be a leader, because I think too many times people do get promoted into a position that is a leadership role, but that doesn't mean they are a leader. I appreciate your definition of leadership. Thank you for sharing that with us.

Ryan: Yes, sir.

Bill: We hear a lot about rural hospital closings. There's a study that suggests that one in three rural hospitals are at risk of closing. It seems like when you hear presentations or read articles about that, states that are in the south are often mentioned, Mississippi in particular, as one of the southern states with major challenges.

One of the reasons I wanted you to be here is to get it from the horse's mouth. What is the state of affairs for rural hospitals in the state of Mississippi?

Ryan: Well, Mississippi, not unlike many states in the south and several states in our country, are facing challenges in our hospital systems. No question about that. I believe you may have seen some recent data published either from CMS or from several consulting groups. Based on the cost report for our critical access hospitals, you could certainly make the claim, and they the claim has been made that 22 out of our 65 hospitals are vulnerable for closure. That's been the big number that's been run with, which is about a third of the hospitals. Simple math will tell you about a third of our hospitals would fall under that risk factor of the possibility of closing.

Of course, any one that knows statistics knows that you have to look at what goes into the data before you can determine what it means. I think in this case that is certainly something we have to look at. What does that mean that 22 of our 65 hospitals are at risk for closure or vulnerable for closure? There are certainly some hospitals in Mississippi that are vulnerable right now. We've had several closures here recently.

One that I might point out is Pioneer Hospital in Newton. This hospital closed, but not because of vulnerability on their cost report but because CMS' reinterpretation of transportation. Critical access hospitals have several factors that determine their eligibility be classified as a critical access hospital. That in includes their distance from other hospitals ad interstate highways. In this case, there was a small stretch of four-lane highway that was built around one city to help with traffic flow. Because there was a one-mile stretch of four-lane highway versus the two-lane highway that existed there before, that one mile-stretch, I think it was even less than one mile, caused that critical access hospital to lose their critical access status.

Bill: Wow.

Ryan: Of course, that's the thing. It's a very unfair thing. There're many hospitals in Mississippi right now that are at risk for closure for that very thing, CMS reinterpretation of guidelines rather than the cost report. That's way more of a fear for us right now than the cost report itself. The reason is because when you look at the operations of hospitals, and our hospital associations have done a great job at looking at the details on this and determining if our hospitals are doing well, why are they doing well. The reason is because the cost report only tells a small picture of what is going on in a hospital. As most of our listeners are probably aware, critical access hospitals in particular receive theoretically one hundred and one percent of reimbursement for cost of their care, which gives them a one percent margin to spend on things that are not allowed on the cost report like advertising and staff development and things like that.

I know you've had previous guests that have mentioned this. Sequestration took two percent right off the top, so they go from one hundred and one percent of reimbursement to ninety-nine percent of reimbursement. Automatically, they lose money on the cost report.

Then several other cuts that have come up, a quarter percent here, half a percent here. In the end, we figure our critical access hospitals are being reimbursed at about 97.5% of their costs.

Bill: Okay.

Ryan: No reasonable person would open a business if you know you're going to lose 2.5% per year, right?

Bill: Right.

Ryan: The big picture, and this is why you see so many hospitals that look like they're bleeding money, is 2.5% of the overall budget of even a small hospital could be millions of dollars.

You have to look deeper than just the numbers. The numbers do show a tragic picture in our future. The hospitals that are doing well, and there are many in Mississippi that are doing well are not just a stand-alone hospital. They are a medical system. They own rural health clinics, swing beds and nursing homes. They have ancillary services like infusion therapy and sleep labs. They have money that comes in as a system, and not just the hospital itself, and that's where the data doesn't show the true picture.

A good example of this is Noxubee General Hospital in Macon. They recently were on a list that Mississippi developed based on cost report data showing that the hospital was in dire risk of closure. But their hospital administrator, Danny McKay, is clearly saying that is simply not the case. The cost report data does show them being, I forget the exact percentage, but it was somewhere around 97.5% cost-based reimbursement. They lose a few percent per year. But that is not their bottom line. That's simply what's publicly reported on the cost report.

Ryan: They actually are doing well. They make money every year. Their employees are not at risk of being laid off because of budget cuts. They're not at risk for closure right now. They're not doing exceptionally well, but most hospitals, even urban well-thought out hospitals, are not doing exceptionally well. They're all facing pressure from ACA, and they're all struggling to keep up with all of the healthcare reform as it is coming down. But they're not about to close either. That's really the state that I see for rural and critical access hospitals in Mississippi.

There's always room for improvement. There're always things they can do to continue to grow and expand and find new sources of revenue. And they are actively searching for that. I believe telehealth is a huge example of that. We are all looking for ways to find suitable reimbursement for services, chronic care management being a great example of that. Overall, our hospitals, they're not failing.

A great example, and Danny mentioned this recently when I spoke to him, our hospitals are like a gas station. A gas station makes a very, very, very thin margin off of gasoline, very, very little. Not even enough to keep the doors open. The reason gas stations are there is because of the convenience store on the inside. You're selling Snickers and chips and soda for sixty-five cents for a Big Gulp cup.

Of course, I hate the fact they sell tobacco and cigarettes, but they do that and make money off it. They make their money off the convenience store, and the gas is just one reason to draw people in. They don't make the money off the gas.

Hospitals are very much the same way. The hospital is your core to get people in, but you're making money off of the convenience store, off of the rural health clinics, off of the nursing home, the other services they provide. If you looked at all the gas stations in Mississippi, you'd say every one of them are about to close based on gasoline profits, but they all do well and they thrive because they find other services they can deliver to meet their customer's needs.

When you look at hospitals like a gas station, it starts to make sense on why they're all staying alive, why they're not closing like everyone's fearing they will. If you boxed out a gas station because of a two-lane highway and say you can no longer have gas, then, yeah, the gas station may close. That's really more of our fear, that CMS' reinterpretation of guidelines based on no really good data. They just decided they wanted to change their mind on something, and now you're talking about hospital closures. Our fear is not necessarily the cost report.

Bill: Understood! I've not heard that gas station analogy before, but I like that. I might be stealing that from you, Ryan.

Ryan: Sure. Well, I stole it from Danny, so feel free.

Bill: Thank you, Ryan. You shared some great information and helped clarify quite a bit on what's really happening, the true story about what's really happening in Mississippi rural hospitals.

You mentioned Danny McKay as one of your rural hospital CEOs. Can you talk about some of the successful rural hospital CEOs that you've come to know and who's being successful and why they're being successful?

Ryan: Sure. We have so many. I can't think of a single hospital administrator in Mississippi that is not exceptional in what they do, all in their own unique way. They all try different things to benefit their facility. They're trying to think outside the box. So many, I really hate to mention certain names and not mention others, but I'll mention a few facilities in particular that I feel are doing some unique things right now and definitely their leadership is one of the reasons.

One that you've probably seen national attention on is in Louisville, Mississippi, one of the poorest counties in the state. The county also has one of the worst education outcomes. Louisville is in Sunflower County in the Mississippi Delta. That is where North Sunflower Medical Center is. North Sunflower and the people in Mississippi are probably tired of hearing about North Sunflower because they're the poster child of what to do at a rural hospital. Given the population of Louisville, they are Medicaid heavy.

North Sunflower Medical Center is one of the rural hospitals that is not going to look exceptionally great on the cost report. But they have some tremendous programs going on. They have a wellness center. They operate clinics. They operate nursing homes. They have of course a great 340B program which is one of those critical things that's helping our hospitals right now. They are investing in the City of Louisville. The hospital itself is helping pharmacies, helping other services that are only quasi-medical at best, helping them to grow to build the entire city back up, increasing the quality of life there. You're starting to look at fresh fruits and vegetables coming back to these towns where the local convenience store is your best source of food, tragically, in these areas. That is a great example of a hospital that is thinking outside the box and using their resources very wisely. Everyone is jumping on board. People will drive to Louisville to come to that facility.

They are also a major leader in chronic care management. They actually have a tele-health program right now for a certain patient population for diabetes and are seeing some extremely strong results with direct patient monitoring.

Another great example is Baptist Medical Center in Leake County, which is in Carthage, Mississippi. They are one of many that has just built a brand-new facility.

What's unique about that facility, like many, is that it is owned by a larger medical center, of course, that being Baptist. They are a gorgeous facility reinvented to meet the direct needs of a population. They're one that you could say is a new facility that has really determined why they want to exist and built the facility around that. Of course, most of our hospitals were built decades ago, and so they were built for services that are no longer needed. We don't need forty patient beds in a city of five thousand people.

You might need five, and you can reinvent the other space for other needs. That would be just one of many examples that is thinking outside the box and trying to reinvent themselves.

There's another hospital that's being built, Hardy Wilson Memorial Hospital in Hazelhurst. Construction is nearing completion soon. It is another hospital that is looking at the demands of their area and reinventing itself to meet those demands.

Bill: Interesting.

Ryan: So many great administrators in Mississippi that are doing good things.

Bill: Those are some interesting things. It's surprising that all the new construction is going on there.

Bill: You mentioned three different facilities there, and you mentioned Danny, our friend with the gas station analogy. You've seen a lot of CEOs in your role as Executive Director of the Mississippi Rural Health Association. You've seen a lot of rural hospital CEOs. You said that they are all great in their own ways. In your opinion, the CEOs that are really making a difference, what would you say their top leadership strengths are?

Ryan: That's a great question. The ones that I know that are widely seen as a great leader in their area do kind of like what I mentioned earlier. They listen to their employees. They empower their employees. That's a huge one in rural health, to feel empowered. There are so few people that move to rural areas, in particular your high-skilled nurse practitioners, physicians, and specialists. If they move to a rural area, they need to feel empowered and really all staff do. If you're sweeping the floors, if you're a technician for one of the pieces of equipment, an IT director, billing and coding staff, you have to feel empowered. You have to feel appreciated. Those administrators that are doing what I would feel is an exceptional job are doing just that.

Ryan: They're not keeping a blind eye, but they are empowering. They check. They show appreciation. They reward that, maybe not financially, although that is a great thing, but they reward it with maybe extra responsibility or extra notoriety in that facility, and it really shows a great effect.

Bill: The top two leadership strengths then that you would consider would be listening and empowering others.

Ryan: Yes.

Bill: Great! Thank you, Ryan. You've seen a lot of CEOs try a lot of different things. What's one of the most unique things that you've seen a rural hospital CEO try that actually worked?

Ryan: One of the most unique things I've seen that worked, I would have to go back to the telehealth example. Telehealth in Mississippi, really throughout the country, is one of those things that everyone gets the concept of but few people are willing to jump off and try it. We have a few people that have jumped off and tried it. North Sunflower is an example. A lot of facilities that have the equipment are just dabbling in it.

Ryan: That takes some risk, though. It takes risk to invest tens or even hundreds of thousands of dollars of equipment to hire staff that can do this. To alter your operation to incorporate an entirely new service. Those that are willing to take the risk and go off in a direction that's almost unknown at this point is something that takes guts. It really takes someone with the mindset that they're willing to trust in what they're hearing and they're willing to go with something they believe and they're told is going to be the future of healthcare.

We are starting to see facilities, more and more of them now, going off into this direction. I think it's going to produce tremendous results for them as reimbursement catches up with telehealth services and the regulations ease just a little bit. I think we're going to see some great results, and I think it's going to be due to the leadership we have right now in trusting in services like this.

Bill: Interesting. Thank you for sharing that. As the Executive Director of the Mississippi Rural Health Association, what are some of the unique things that your organization is doing to advance rural health in the state of Mississippi?

Ryan: We've really worked hard to grow in the direction that our members need us to grow. We serve most of the hospitals, the rural health clinics, several FQHCs, other rural providers that don't necessarily fall into those categories, students and universities. We've got the entire gambit; eleven-hundred members in total right now. We really try to fit the needs of everyone.

For hospitals and clinics, we're trying to incorporate quality reporting measures right now to where they can begin to report quality if they're not already required to. If they are required to, trying to help them with training and education and understanding MIPS and MACRA and all of the new reporting systems that are evolving. For those that are not required, we're trying to develop quality tools that they can experiment with almost like a sandbox. We developed the nation's first rural health professional credential designed for people to really show on their resume that they have distinct experience with rural health and to really give them notoriety for that. It's called the Mississippi Rural Health Fellow.

Bill: How do they get that, Ryan?

Ryan: The requirement is they have to have at least three years of rural specific experience. They have to have completed up to seventy-five hours of professional education over the past three years. That could be both with our association, and right now, we allow it with other associations as well.

They also have to complete a quality improvement project in their community. We're pretty flexible on what that looks like depending on what their professional role is, but they have to complete a quality improvement project. We do have a small fee that participants pay, $100 per year, for three years, to receive this certification. Once earned, they are able to put the letters NRHA after their name. They are able to show that they are a "rural health professional." It's been very well-received.

Bill: Very cool! I've not heard of this program before.

Ryan: Then there are other things that we're doing. We lead projects throughout the state with training and education. We advocate and lobby for our members with state-based and national legislation. The national legislation pretty well lines up with what the American Hospital Association and of course the National World Health Association are doing. State-based, there's a variety of things we work on. There is a lot more that we do that just tries to meet the direct needs of our members.

Bill: That's great. Thank you for sharing that, and thank you for your work in the state of Mississippi.

Bill: What do you see, not just in Mississippi, but what do you see is the future for rural health?

Ryan: When I think of rural health, I think of a time that our association secretary, Zack Gala, came up with. Zack is the Vice President for Children's International Medical Group, which stretches across several states. He also served in the Louisiana Rural Health Association. Zack has grown this passion for the concept called "one rural." In fact, he's even developed a hashtag, #OneRural. They've been using that hashtag recently with the Louisiana flooding. It has been such a great story of the Louisiana Rural Health Association helping the rural health clinics in their communities to rebuild and to try to get back on their feet as quickly as possible. This hashtag has really grown out of this.

When I think of what excites me about rural and what the future is in the rural community that we have, it's not just a rural association, but the individuals, the people, everyone who lives in rural. You see a disaster, and you immediately see people get out to help their neighbor. This is a southern kind of strap on your boots and go to work. You see that over and over again. It's the people in these rural areas that are drivers behind that. We are a committee.

We believe in each other. We put competition to the side. We become brothers and sisters, standing hand-in-hand, working together.

That's what excites me about the future of rural. There are still going to be challenges. There're going to be things that are less advantageous for us, even though quality measures are just as high and our reimbursement for services are far lower than urban. We always seem to get behind the eight ball when it comes to the perception of rural, yet when everyone thinks of who they believe in, it's always rural. They always come back to the roots they came from. And that, I believe, is going to be the future of our country.

People are going to realize that rural health, or rural matters in general, are the core of our country. It's where we were founded. It's where we belong. I believe that that's going to translate into a greater understanding of why rural healthcare is just as high quality as urban healthcare, why people are going to want to move back to rural areas to get away from the hustle and bustle of city life. Why our communities, our rural communities, are going to continue to thrive, continue to do well. We're going to continue to have industry moving to rural areas. Education is going to continue to improve. I have a great outlook when it comes to not just rural health but rural communities in general.

Bill: Ryan, I can hear the passion in your voice, and I thank you so much for sharing your expertise, your thoughts, your observations and experiences in rural health. Thank you for all the good work you and all the other rural healthcare providers in the state of Mississippi are doing.

Marc Augsburger

Marc Augsburger is the President and CEO of Caro Community Hospital in Caro, Michigan. Learning is a running theme through the interview as Marc talks about how effective rural health leaders are always learning, whether it is form our mistakes or interns. The conversation also focuses on the importance of open conversations and building relationship within a healthcare facility. This and much more is explored in the following interview.

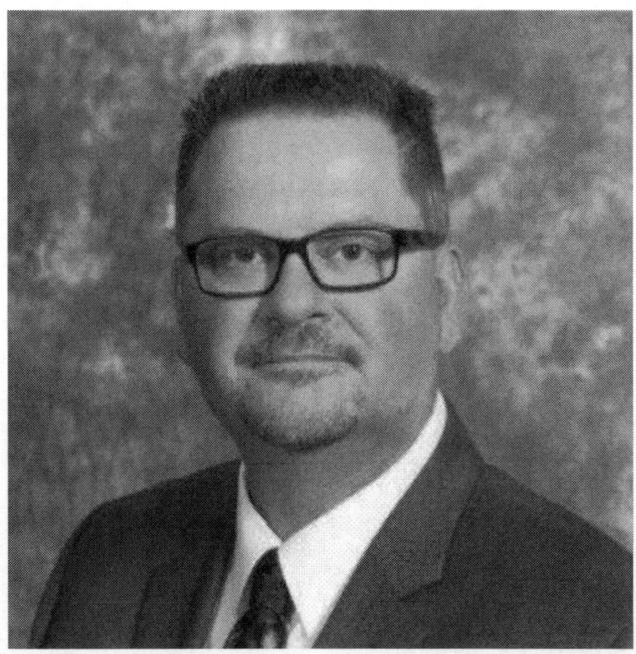

Bill: Marc Augsburger was born and raised in Northwest Ohio, and graduated from nursing school in 1988 with an Associate's Degree in Nursing. From there, he went on to earn his Bachelor of Science in Nursing and an MBA with an emphasis in healthcare. He's primarily worked in critical care and emergency nursing prior to moving into a senior role as a hospital administrator. He was the CEO of Horn Memorial Hospital in Ida Grove, Iowa, and then assumed the CEO role at Caro Community Hospital in Caro, Michigan, in April of 2013. He just celebrated his three-year anniversary there.

Marc: Yes, I did!

Bill: He's been married to Melissa since 1999 and they have two daughters, Greta and Molly.

Let's get right into it, Marc. I have a lot of questions that I want to ask, but first, why did you choose healthcare for a career?

Marc: I have been very interested in healthcare since I was a little boy. Having had some illnesses when I was young that required a lot of physician visits and some hospitalizations, I had a great early experience on what healthcare is, and that seemed to drive my interest in heading into the healthcare realm. I love being with people. I love talking to people and meeting with them. I think that great thing s like palliative care that we have today is a great opportunity. Helping educate people and keeping them healthy drove my interest back then and continues to motivate me today.

Bill: One thing that you and I both share is that at a young age, we both had an inclination that we were interested in healthcare. I think that both of us, our first jobs, our first real jobs in healthcare, were as nurses' aids in a hospital. Is that right?

Marc: That's correct. When I was still in high school, I started as a candy striper at the small critical access hospital in Bluffton, Ohio. I was a volunteer and then a nursing assistant while I was going through my initial Associate's Degree. Those really were forming years.

Bill: Yes. That was a great way to break into healthcare.

Marc: That's right.

Bill: Why rural health?

Marc: I really have been interested all my life in rural healthcare because, growing up, Bluffton, Ohio, was a city of about 4,200 people. Now, Caro, Michigan, the city I currently reside in and where my hospital is, also has 4,200 residents. It's sort of like being back home. I've certainly lived in much larger cities. I have worked at a large 700 bed hospital. I really like the opportunity that rural health provides, that niche of care that we offer. While we may not do all of the big cases, we do a great job in rural America with minor to moderate care to keep our residents local. We really like to keep them from having to drive 40 plus miles into a city or much further for care, especially to see a specialist. I like to bring the specialist here instead, and if we need something big we go elsewhere. You can't beat rural health.

Bill: Thank you, Marc. I appreciate what you are doing. We need people like you in rural health who have that passion. Marc, how do you define leadership?

Marc: Leadership to me is an opportunity to guide staff to do the right thing. I like to go back to the statement, do unto others what you would want done to or for you, or a family member. Leadership to me is all about guiding and mentoring people to make good decisions and provide an opportunity to feel good about what they're doing. Of course, we all make mistakes. A good leader will always learn from those mistakes and help teach others how to avoid those same kinds of issues in the future.

Bill: One thing I find interesting about your definition of leadership is the idea of guiding and mentoring others. Did you have a mentor?

Marc: I did. I've had a number of mentors. First in nursing. I had a director of an emergency department that, boy, I sort of idolized. Everything she did and the way she led us and helped mentor and teach just seemed like the right thing to do. It was always a win-win situation. While earning my Master's Degree, I really had a couple of either COOs or CEOs that I took a real liking to. They were very interested in helping me pursue my goals and make it work for the best. It's just amazing how much you can learn with somebody that's interested in mentoring others.

Bill: It's very powerful. The other question I want to ask you, particularly about mentoring, since you make it a point to mentor others as part of your leadership definition is this; it's easy to recognize the benefit as the recipient of mentoring, being the mentee. What has been your experience as a mentor? What have been the rewards to you when you mentor others?

Marc: Actually, that question rings home right now. I'm working with someone pursuing their bachelor's right now in healthcare management. We're doing a 120-hour internship, and internship of course is a big part of the program. I think that not only do they gain wisdom from the things that I and other members of my executive leadership team do, but I learn every single day from those mentoring opportunities as well. Every day, we don't necessarily top and think about what we're doing and why. We are just doing our jobs. It seems natural to just keep moving forward with our daily routine.

When you are mentoring someone, whether it's a distant occasional mentorship or constant like the internship right now, you step back and think a lot more about what you're doing. You think about things like all of the acronyms we use. You step back and go, "Gosh. There's a lot more to my job than I even think about." It's just hugely refreshing and rewarding for both the mentor and the mentee.

Bill: The power of serving others is tremendous on both sides. Thank you for sharing that. Marc, what would you say is your top leadership strength?

Marc: My top leadership talent is an ability to have great open conversations with any healthcare provider. It doesn't matter if it's my front-line staff, a physician, or a mid-level providing surgical services for our patients. We really like to keep the lines of communication open. I fully believe in making rounds. I can't say enough how important that is. I know that we often don't get the opportunity to do that every day. Certainly, touching base with your departments, getting to know them, taking the necessary time to meet with them. It doesn't matter if it's early in the morning or late in the evening. Making sure that we're all doing the right thing and having critical conversations are extremely important.

Bill: Effective communication is an important part of leadership. These conversations, open conversations, was that something that was intentional on your part? Have you honed that skill through intention? How have you evolved as a leader with that skill?

Marc: Absolutely. In my readings and literature research and watching other very successful leaders in healthcare, one of the commonalities amongst most all of them is the ability to get to know your staff, or at least get out and make yourself visible. There are numerous organizations where people don't even know who the CEO is. Maybe they have an idea from the picture, they've seen every once in a while. There's nothing better than getting to the laboratory, getting to nursing, the pharmacy, materials management, or housekeeping. You really want to take a look at their jobs. Job shadowing is one of the best things a CEO can do. We need to know what kind of energies and efforts are required for the job and that they're putting into their job. Odds are, that is more important than they know what you're doing. There's nothing better than a great team working together.

Bill: Thank you. What's something unique that you've done as the CEO that's worked?

Marc: While it may not sound horribly important to everyone, I'll go back again to making rounds as often as possible. This provides the opportunity to get to know your staff better really puts you in a better position to gain the support of your staff. You want to acknowledge them in their work areas. Calling a staff member by name is really important. It gives that extra sense of, "Wow, the boss really does know who I am and cares about me. That's great." Get to know a little something about their family. That's always something good. Ask questions; get to know who the kids are.

One of the things that I've done that I learned from a great mentor of mine was that, for every employee's child ten and under for their birthday, I actually send them a birthday card and stick a $2 bill in it.

Now, as you probably know, there are a lot of kids that have never seen a $2 bill. In fact, I have had some parents come back and say, "You know, my kid came to me and said, is this real? Was this a fake thing that they put in?" It's like, "No, no. That's real money." That's one of those special things. With every card that goes out, I always thank them for letting their mom or dad come to work. That's really important because in the summer, a lot of times kids would like for their parent to be able to stay home, but they need to go to work. There's nothing better than saying thanks for letting your mom and dad get up and come to work. It's just a lot of fun. It is so much appreciated by the children, and the employees just think it's great too. I'm just proud to have that piece with them.

Bill: Absolutely. That is great. I love the $2 bill idea. Thank you, Marc, for what you've shared so far.

We like to talk about things we've done that work, but it's also important to talk about things that we've tried that don't necessarily turn out the way we want. In fact, sometimes, we can even learn from those things. Can you share something that you tried that didn't work or didn't turn out the way you planned?

Marc: This is a little bit of a tough one because looking at if from the front-end, you might say, this should not have happened. I worked with a company in the past that was an emergency department placement company for the physicians. One of the things that never happened was that we were never able to interview or speak with the new emergency department physician staff that were coming in. While that may seem sort of common place, one of the things that I found is that without that initial touch to get to know someone in an interview type process, you have no idea if the staff person that's coming in is going to feel awkward in our facility or if we're going to feel awkward with them. We just don't know what kind of standards that a person will have. Certainly, you would never think of placing an employee in your facility, let alone a physician, without having an interview to make sure they're going to be a good fit.

That could be a disaster. I had a couple of people that, while great practitioners, it just didn't work. We don't practice quite the same as a big city facility. We might not have some of the same equipment. We obviously have very talented staff, so that could be equal. It simply didn't work and I don't want that kind of thing to happen anymore. I always set up some sort of a meet and greet prior to letting them come into work at our facility, and it's been nothing but a win-win since that change started going on a number of years ago.

Bill: Good point, and good lesson. That is a tough lesson, but good way of dealing with it.

Marc, this is the second hospital where you've been the CEO. You've worked in nursing and you've worked in management. In your opinion, what do rural health leaders need to do differently?

Marc: I am going to go back to my earlier comments on making rounds. A really important aspect of making rounds is that it allows you to get to know our staff. I have worked in large facilities and realize that in a large facility, there are way too many employees to get to know all of them. A place with hundreds of employees, there's no way that you can get to know each of them as individually as you can in a position like mine in a rural setting. In rural healthcare, we are all about the family. We are family that often take care of our own and other family members.

We're taking care of the people in the community that are often interrelated in the community. They live in the community that we serve and everybody knows each other. Some of the things that we like to do are again, getting to know the staff. That allows us to work with each other more efficiently and more effectively. We set up tickets to hockey or baseball games for us to go to as a hospital family. We really need to show our staff that we are a leader that cares about them and their family. I just can't say how important that is in rural healthcare.

Bill: That's nice, and growing up in the small town myself, similar to you, it is true. Everybody knows everybody. Working at the hospital, as well as in the community, is very important.

One in three rural hospitals have been identified as being at risk of closing in our country, which is pretty scary. It sounds like you're doing some exciting things that are innovative that are making your organization successful. I have got two questions in one to ask. What excites you the most about the future of rural health, and the flip side of that, what scares you the most about the future of rural health?

Marc: The first thing I'd say Bill, is that, I absolutely love my job. I like getting up and coming to work every day. Everybody has a bad day, but I can't say enough about how great the people are to work with here. However, as you talk about on the scary side, there are a lot of challenges that lie ahead. The unknown is both the most appealing and the scariest part of my job. I really think that critical access hospitals are here to stay. It certainly would be political suicide in my estimation to let this valuable piece of the healthcare industry for rural America go away. We've got to have rural hospitals and certainly critical access hospitals and other federally designated programs to help. Frontier areas are extremely important, and healthcare in America just couldn't go on without that. However, I do believe that cost cut threats are real. They're here to stay.

We definitely need to remain on our toes and preserve the rural healthcare that America needs. What we do know is that a focus on health and wellness are what we need to be practicing first and foremost. It makes sense to keep people out of the hospital. But hospitals are here to stay. too. No matter what, no matter how healthy we make people, there's certainly always going to be illness and care that's going to need to be provided. I do believe though, without a doubt, that more great technology is in store for us, and we do have some more cures coming ahead for dreaded diseases. I think another new exciting aspect of healthcare is that we are moving at light speed. I don't see that stopping anytime soon.

Bill: Thank you for sharing your perspective Marc. What kind of benefits have you experienced when working with a larger facility?

Marc: The great thing about being a rural healthcare facility is that, we always have partners around. Some obviously fit our culture more than others. What we can glean from them is additional knowledge on maybe some new technology, as well as experiences that some of the staff have had. I can't say enough about the number of the regional hospitals that we work with. Their interest in coming out to share their knowledge and experiences with us can be quite beneficial. Sometimes they have some great cost cutting ideas that maybe we haven't thought of or we might not be able to do on our own. That synergy, of large and small hospitals working together works best for American healthcare.

Bill: Interesting. Thank you. As we discussed earlier, we both share the experience of starting out as nurses' aides, and we both agree, that background was valuable for both of us. It does provide you with a broad perspective. You've been a nurse's aide. You've been a nurse with an Associate's Degree, a nurse with a Bachelor of Science Degree, and a Master's Degree in Business. How does all the experience that you have in healthcare, both at work and academically, help you be a better hospital CEO? How does it help you be a better leader?

Marc: I really think, Bill, that the knowledge and ability to have worked hands on with patients and to see their pain, to see their illness, then to see them getting better, really helped to paint a picture and better understanding as the CEO of what all of my staff are doing. It takes everyone. When I was working as a registered nurse, it didn't matter if it was in surgery, the emergency department, or ICU, everybody worked as a collaborative team. I worked with all of the therapist, sometimes it was with physical

therapy or occupational therapy, or housekeeping, the lab, or radiology. I really got a good sense of what people's jobs were and how they worked with each other. Then, tie that together with the education I received when pursuing and earning my MBA, it just gave
me great business knowledge acumen that you don't necessarily get from a nursing degree. You start to get introduced to some of those pieces, and even working as a floor nurse or in a management role, you get some pieces of that, but I tell you what, throwing that together with the MBA really gives you a very well-rounded view of what's going on in your facility and with healthcare.

Bill: If you had it to do all over again, would you choose a leadership path in healthcare?

Marc: I absolutely would! I certainly liked working with patients. Again, it's that whole interaction that I think I talked about early on; getting to know and work with people, that passionate piece. I get to do that same kind of thing in my role today. I still get to see family. Again, making rounds, you get to talk to the staff. You get to talk to patients, their loved ones and family. It's great to work with a bunch of other leaders who have great experiences and know what they're doing. I wouldn't give up my leadership role at all. It's just a culmination of all my experiences put into one, and I'm hoping to continue to keep my facilities doing a great job.

Bill: Marc, thank you. I have no doubt that you'll be able to do that. Thank you so much for sharing your experiences, your thoughts and your observations on rural health.

Dr. David Swenson

Dr. David Swenson has a unique take on rural health. Dr. Swenson is the director of the MBA in Rural healthcare program at the College of St. Scholastica, the only MBA program focused on rural health leadership. In our conversation, he talks through the unique aspects of the program. Further, we delve into the strengths and weaknesses of rural health leadership as a whole, as well as the ups and downs that come with that responsibility.

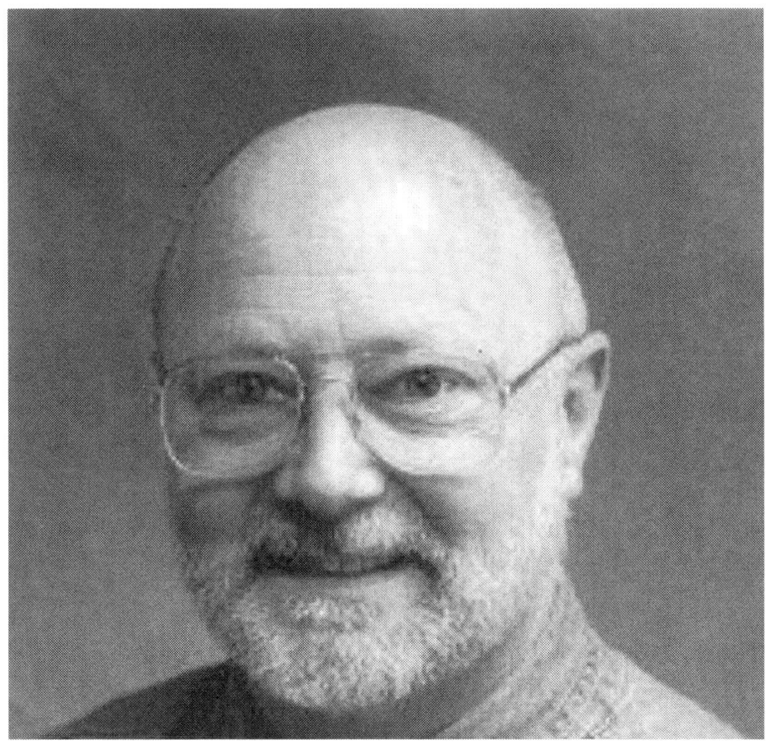

Bill: Dr. David Swenson is the director of the MBA in Rural Healthcare program at the College of St. Scholastica, in Duluth, MN. This is the only US college to focus exclusively on rural healthcare leadership. David has been in the healthcare field for nearly 30 years in multiple roles, as a psychologist, a health educator, a mental health administrator in Missouri, Wisconsin, and Minnesota.

What is your definition of leadership, Dave?

David: I knew you were going to ask about that. That's a hard question in so many ways. I remember I was designing a leadership course several years ago, and I was going through the literature. One of the places that I found said there are about 500 different definitions of leadership in the literature. It kind of depends, you can pick and choose. The one that I really like, and I use it quite often, is getting things done through people. This definition, I think, is important because it's not just one vision and strategy that are important, but I think leadership is working with people and inspiring them to work through change.

Bill: That's great. And I like the simplicity of that and the simplicity of getting things done through other people. A simple statement, a complex concept.

David: I think there's also an interesting distinction between management and leadership. We often think of management as also working with people, but it tends to look at the status quo; what's already operating, what's going on, how can we make that more efficient? Whereas leaders are more in the role, instead of looking at the way things are, they look at what could be. They look at the horizon. They look at the change that is going to be imminent, and how can they prepare their organization to adapt and survive in that emerging environment.

Actually, you need both of those roles, managers and leaders: managers to stabilize, leaders to shake things up. It's really important they understand each other's roles and how to work together, but at the same time I have to say that there is tremendous overlap between managers and leaders. Many managers are involved in the change process themselves. We don't really have a terrific definition, nor do we have a clear definition of the roles of each of them. They are a little muddled together, but as long as we can see that they're complementary, and that leadership is primarily involved with change, then I think that makes sense.

Bill: That's an important distinction to make, and I appreciate you making it. Thank you.

You've had a variety of roles in healthcare; you're a psychologist; you're an educator; and you're a mental health administrator. You've spent almost 50 years in healthcare. Why did you choose healthcare as a career path?

David: That's a good question too. I was even a career counselor in my early years as a doctoral student, and I'd like to say that I've been extremely planful in my career. I have always looked around to see what kind of jobs are needed. I look at my skill set and what I need to develop to fill that gap. I have had a lot of plans, but I guess my point is, that all the careers that I've had, all the different positions and roles that I've had, have almost never been by plan.

I've been in a lot of different situations. It really comes down to my philosophy. I like paying attention to what's happening in the system at the time, therefore, many of the roles that I take on have been emergent roles; I was there, I saw the opportunity and I moved into that. All the positions that I've had have been once based on something that I believe in, something that I think is important. Seeing people in need, seeing a crisis, helping people solve problems and the role and the title have sort of been secondary to the jumping into that.

Bill: Interesting. Thank you for sharing that.

You know a tremendous amount about leadership. You've already demonstrated that by what you've shared so far, and you've had different leadership positions, and you continue to be a leader today. You even teach leadership. For you specifically, as a leader, what do you feel your top leadership strength is?

David: I tend to think of things in clusters and groups, how different factors come together to produce something. So, I don't know if I can give you the number one top thing, but there are maybe two or three different qualities or characteristics that I think characterize most of what I do.

The first one is, I tend to be pretty reflective. I can be decisive. I'm often described by my colleagues as really driven and assertive, and I think that's characteristic of me too, but every once in a while, I really believe it's essential to step back and see what I'm doing and where I'm going. If I'm in a team meeting, I want to step back and observe the process for a while. If I'm in a strategy meeting, I want to step back and see if other people are engaged, or if I'm just talking by myself. I think that reflective qualities of listening, observing, and understanding, those are really important. As leaders, we can get a, what we used to say when I lived in Missouri, we can get a bug under the hood and it just kind of drives you. I think that's true, we can get enthusiastic and feel driven about things, but we have to stop and step back a little bit and see if what we're doing is making sense and if other people are on board.

Related to that is an insatiable curiosity. I'm absolutely fascinated about why people do what they do and how they think. I'm also a forensics psychologist. I think of some of the distasteful people I've worked with in the criminal justice system, such as psychopaths, and I like to understand how they can put the world together in a way that justifies their behavior.

Bill: Interesting.

David: But frankly it's no different when as an organization development consultant, I go into a group of executives and I try to understand how they view their discipline in the business world and the marketplace they're in, that drives their decisions.

That curiosity is really important. It leads us to ask questions, and more important, it leads us to listen to people. Instead of grabbing onto an idea and running with it, it allows us to really understand what people are saying and what's behind that. The last point I will make is systems thinking. I'll probably talk a little bit more about this in regard to some of your other questions, but that's one of the areas that I think really captures the way that I think about things. I don't look at problems or issues in isolation. It's easy to do that, because then you can kind of capture it and you can put parameters on it. But most of the time things are kind of messy. They're ambiguous to us. There are a lot of different factors that come together to create a problem. When we make a decision, often there are consequences that we haven't considered.

I tend to characterize my leadership style as one that uses systems thinking. I think that combination of reflection and curiosity and systems thinking, that combination probably captures more of the way I go about things.

Bill: Interesting concept! You mentioned earlier when you were talking about choosing healthcare as a career, you listened to the systems to figure what was important and what was emerging so systems thinking seems to be a recurring theme with you, Dave.

David: It is!

Bill: You've worked with quite a few leaders in rural health. You have seen quite a variety of leaders and multiple experiences on differing topics with different leaders in rural health. Can you provide any examples or talk about some leadership that you've experienced in rural health, that you've felt like was exceptional leadership?

David: Yes! I think there are a couple of qualities that really stand out with many of the rural leaders that I've worked with and spoken to. The first is their level of conviction. Working in rural healthcare is really a challenge. You don't have as many resources, you work with a somewhat different constellation of problems than you do in urban areas. I think many people simply don't have the background for that kind of exposure, so they struggle through it, but they stick with it. That conviction is something that always impresses me with people in rural healthcare. Related to that is creativity. Common solutions don't necessarily work with some of the uncommon problems that emerge in rural healthcare.

One of my colleagues that I've worked with many years, Terry Hill, was a former executive director of the National Rural Health Resource Center, based here in Duluth. Terry and I have worked together for many years. I think he's been in the field for almost 40 years now, and he's worked in almost all 50 states. He's written lots of articles and led several national demonstration projects in rural health. He's just a remarkable person with untiring energy.

What he does that I so admire are his listening skills. He draws people out. He tries to understand what it is that is going on. He uses his systems approach. "Does this seem to account to what you're experiencing? Is this where the problem is?" And he helps them try to understand how the way they've structured work and how they go about thinking about the problem may actually be the way in which they keep themselves from solving it. It involves a lot of listening, communication, a great deal of empathy, persistence, and the ability to communicate clearly what you hear people saying, and then presenting that back to them as some leverage points they can change. I just admire that style, and he's been doing it for so long, and he's worked with people at a variety of levels across the country. That's the kind of versatility that I'm very impressed with.

Bill: I met Terry the same time I met you. I've had a couple of conversations with Terry, and what he has done is very impressive. Hopefully, he'll be a future guest here as well.

David: I hope so.

Bill: Were there any other examples you wanted to share of exceptional leadership?

David: Yes! Tim Rice at the Lakewood Health Systems in Staples, Minnesota. Staples is a very small community, and Tim has ended up being a nationally recognized figure in rural health for his system. He has many of the same characteristics that Terry does. He's also interestingly one of the graduates from our earlier MBA program and he is putting to practice many of the things that we're now talking about in our Rural Health MBA program.

Dave: He does the same thing. He's engaging; he's inclusive; he brings people together. While he has his own ideas, you can't take your own ideas and push them off on people. You have to draw people out, find out what they need, and find the connection between the change that's needed, and understand why people resist change. Tim is particularly strong at that.

Bill: What is one of the more important leadership skills that you often find lacking in rural health leaders?

David: I'm afraid I'm going to have to come back to systems thinking again.

Bill: You said that would be a recurring theme.

David: It is! It is! I beat the drum about that one a lot. Primarily because I don't find it as widely used as I think would be helpful. In our culture, we tend to think about things in somewhat linear, and I guess, sort of isolated or siloed ways. When we have a problem, we define the problem and put parameters around it. We solve for that problem. We come up with a solution. We implement it. We feel pretty good about it. The problem is, in many cases, we don't think about the constellation of forces that have produced the problem in the first place. In some cases, even worse, we don't think about the impact of our decision downstream. If we think about organizations and think of our actions a little bit like a stream, I think that's important, because there are a lot of streams that come into it, and there are a lot of tributaries that run off of it.

We don't think about those ripple effects when we make decisions. We have good people who are bright people. They are very involved. They think the problem through. But if they don't consider what those downstream effects might be, then what is the solution in one context at one time, may in fact be another problem or even a worse problem at some other part of the organization, or in the community image, or someplace else.

There's a good example of that in pharmaceuticals. Antibiotics, as we all know, have been tremendous in reducing infection rates and very powerful in maintaining health as a medical intervention. But the enthusiasm over those has led to feeding livestock and to people abusing antibiotics, so that now we have antibiotic resistant diseases that are really serious. They do not have the same kind of treatments available. In the same way, we tend to look at a solution and we implement that without considering what the consequences are.

Edward Tenner, a few years ago, had a book called "Revenge Effects" that really had an impact on me. I think Tenner's book on Revenge Effects and Peter Senge's book on the Fifth Discipline, which was on systems thinking, both of those really had impact on me, so that when I do my consulting, and certainly when I do my own practice and my own teaching, I tend to not look at problems in silos, but I start looking for connections. When I make a decision, I look at the impact of that decision downstream as much as I can.

It's not like systems thinking is that alien to us. In physiology, for example, we certainly understand if we affect one physiological system, it often will have a ripple effect through other parts of the system in human behavior. Sometimes cognition and emotion. Things are really connected and we understand that in physiology. What we need to do is also understand that in our organizations and our communities in rural health, so that when we tweak something in one area, it can have a beneficial or it can sometimes have adverse effects elsewhere.

I think we do a lot of systems thinking, but we don't recognize it as such. The Baldrige Leadership Award, which now covers healthcare and looks for extraordinary leadership in systems thinking. The Triple Aim, the Balanced Scorecard, all these are pretty good examples of systems thinking.

But we need to practice it in day to day for it to work as well.

Bill: Great point!

Talk about the MBA program that you have created.

David: About six years ago, maybe a little longer than that, Terry Hill and I used to get together every once in a while, for a cup of coffee or a beer after work.

We would talk about some of the different issues that we'd run across in our daily work consulting and teaching. Healthcare continued to be the key focus, which both of us are so committed to and interested in. After a couple of years of that, we decided to form what we now call the Lake Superior Core Systems Thinking Group. We brought together anywhere from eight to as many as thirty different professionals from different fields. We would meet once a month. We talked about issues like how do you deliver healthcare to rural veterans. How do we understand the increase in chemical abuse in rural communities? What are the dynamics that give rise to school violence and school shootings? We are in our fifth year now of that.

Most of what we've come up with are some interesting perspectives on change and involving leaders in the community to some of those health issues. As leaders in rural health, it's not just our organizations that we're involved in as leaders, it's the communities. We have to have a community base for the changes that we want. Out of those conversations, Terry and I started thinking, there are a lot of well-intentioned people who have expert knowledge in healthcare. We have physicians and nurses and PAs, social workers, occupational therapists, a whole range of healthcare people, and they have expert knowledge in their field. So much though, that many of them move into administrative positions, because they see the changes that are important.

The catch is, most of them don't have a background in business, and increasingly, this is a healthcare business. It involves understanding finance and marketing, and all sorts of things. A good example of that marketing is somewhere around 60% of the people in our rural communities go outside of those rural communities for healthcare that is actually provided in those communities.

I think that's a good example of inefficient marketing. This is an example of a lack of skills that can be learned and can be applied in those settings.

That's sort of the origin of it. We got together with Randy Zimmerman, who is Director of our Graduate Studies at the College of St. Scholastica in Duluth. We looked at our current MBA program, and we realized that a regular MBA is not what we were looking for. I actually went online because part of what I do is marketing as well. I was looking at who our competitors might be, and what was the status of MBAs in rural healthcare. I know you mentioned this at the beginning, we turned out to be the only program that exclusively focuses on rural healthcare. I was amazed by that.

Bill: Yes. I did research myself, and yours was the only program I could find exclusive to rural health.

David: I looked at about 72 different programs, and I thought they were all very good programs too. They were MBA's in healthcare, but it's a broad range of healthcare. In fact, the only other program that I could find is in India, on rural healthcare. They have a few courses, maybe they have a track, but entire curriculum, there's none devoted to it. That seemed like a real opportunity for us to fill that gap. And that's what we've done.

The final thing I did, was to put together a board of directors of people who have national reputations and good levels of experience in rural healthcare. I went through the literature, I asked those people, and we built a curriculum in a little bit of a different way. A lot of times in curricula you would, for example, take a finance course. Fine, we know what goes into a finance course, we'll have a finance course and a marketing course, a program evaluation course, and healthcare administration course, and we'll search the literature and we'll see what's popular, and we'll put that into it. We decided not to do that.

Instead what we did was to ask people on the front lines and at the top of the healthcare organizations, "What do you wish you would have known when you went into this field? How is the field changing, and what are the skills that you really need to have now?" We started clustering together the kinds of skills and behaviors and understandings that people expressed, and sure enough, there were some that clustered under finance and some that clustered under marketing and human resources. What we did was build our curriculum from the ground up, not the top down. That, I believe, insures that what we're looking at is a very applied kind of a program.

My goal is for people to come out of each class session, probably each class session may be a bit much, but come out of every class session and say, "I know something now I didn't know before, and I can go back to work tomorrow, and I can understand things a little differently, and may even be able to do something differently." That's our goal with the program as well.

We were originally a liberal arts school. The characterization was, "We are scholars with the sleeves rolled up." I really liked that image. That's still sort of the image I have. We have professionals, but professionals who are right down there in the trenches. They understand what it's like on the front lines, and at the same time, they understand theory and they understand literature, and they can take the big picture and apply that right at the ground level.

That's been my goal, and that's how we built the program.

Bill: That's a very pragmatic approach, like you said, so someone can take what they learned today, and apply it tomorrow.

David: Exactly.

Bill: That's very interesting.

Getting a program up and running like this, it seems like an insurmountable task to me, but obviously you've done it, and done it quite well. What has been one of the surprises in getting the program up and running? Both the good and the bad.

David: I don't know if it's the bad, but what I was most surprised about is that there were really no other programs that emphasized rural health to the degree that we were proposing. There were a lot of excellent programs around the country, and they maybe had a course or two.

I know medical education, actually education in most of the professions, has a lot of information to cram into it. In fact, that's one of the challenges that I see in higher education right now. In order to compete in the marketplace, we have to make all of our programs seem more and more attractive and more and more convenient. Part of what's happening is that we're condensing many courses into shorter periods of time.

Frankly, if some people don't see rural healthcare as important, they may have only a single course in it. Our objective is to prepare people to specifically go into the rural health arena, but I also have to say, we've got some students who work in the urban areas, they work with large healthcare systems. Part of why they want to get this background in rural health is because they're working on connecting those rural health systems with the larger urban systems.

Bill: Interesting.

David: I think that's important too.

Bill: Absolutely!

David: The other positive thing is as we look at the students who are coming into our MBA program. They represent just about every healthcare discipline you can imagine. We need to work as colleagues, and we need to collaborate with people from different backgrounds, not be siloed just in our own professions. The diversity of the students coming into our MBA is something I just feel wonderful about.

Bill: From all different service lines within the healthcare system?

David: Yes! About half, maybe two thirds are already healthcare managers and they want to update their skills. But we have people in nursing and financial specialists, rehab specialists, mental health people, pharmacists, radiology, medical technology, even an attorney. Really, quite a diverse group.

Bill: Very interesting. You're preparing the leaders for tomorrow, or the leaders for today, for that matter, for rural health. As we all know, rural health has some major challenges that we're up against today with one in three rural hospitals have been identified as at risk of failing.

Dave, what scares you the most about the future of rural health?

David: There's a lot that scares me. I think probably the biggest one is that we will make changes in healthcare, but I'm afraid they may be too late for a lot of people. We need those changes now. There are people suffering now, who are unable to find transportation out of their communities. We have, as you mentioned, critical access hospitals that are closing. We have a scarcity of physicians, but I think we'll probably find some ways around that. Often, we, as a people, wait until the crisis occurs, and when it's bad enough, then we fix it. In the meantime, a lot of people suffer for it. I think that's probably my biggest worry.

Peter Senge, the systems specialist I mentioned earlier, had a particular saying. He said that "Every system delivers exactly what it's designed to do." So, if we have consequences we don't like now, it's probably a result of the structure that we have created. The new population approach and value approach that we're working on in healthcare is going to change that. But it's going to take a while. We're moving in the right direction. We need to find leaders who are going to be active and experiment in new designs and be able to conduct research to get evidence to show how much more effective it is. We need to have people to influence our legislators and decision makers. We need to have leaders in healthcare, not just stay within their organizations, but be much more active in their communities to mobilize that kind of action. I'm hopeful, but I think what scares me is that it's going to take time for all that to occur.

Bill: Yes. Rural health is so complex and such a challenge. What excites you the most about the future of rural health?

David: I think it's all the people that I meet. It's people in the communities who are not in the healthcare system, and they want something different; they want something better. They're a very vocal group. I think that's probably what excites me most, because if change is going to occur, it's going to occur through people.

Let me give an example of an issue. The one issue that has been catching my interest recently is climate change, and the impact of climate change on health and human services. There's still about 30% of the American population in some areas, about 50% of politicians, maybe more, who just don't buy into that yet. What I see is a healthcare crisis in the offing if we don't pay attention to that.

I'm in Minnesota, and when we talked about Lyme disease years ago, we talked about that in Lyme, Connecticut, and now Lyme disease and ticks are pretty much all over the state of Minnesota. Primarily due to warmer weather and the winters not killing them off. I don't want to go into a tirade about climate change, but it's simply a good example of how large-scale changes can impact health and human services. Health, and also, the delivery of those services. We are talking as much about that. What excites me is when we get people who are vocal about it, and they do have strong convictions, and they have evidence, and they take the time and the energy to bring it to people who are the decision makers.

Bill: I love that. People do make the difference and people like you, Dave, are making a huge difference in rural health today.

Dave, I truly want to thank you for sharing your thoughts and observations in your experience in rural health.

Janelle Ali-Dinar, Ph.D.

In the fourteenth episode of *Rural Health Leadership Radio™*, I interviewed Janelle Ali-Dinar, PhD. Our conversation covers aspects of rural health and leadership from the need to inspire, transform, and adapt to changes in health care, to Ali-Dinar's work creating the "We Are One" campaign which works to help everyone in a healthcare facility work together to make the system run smoother. We examine the need for strategic planning and forward thinking in rural healthcare and much more in the interview that follows.

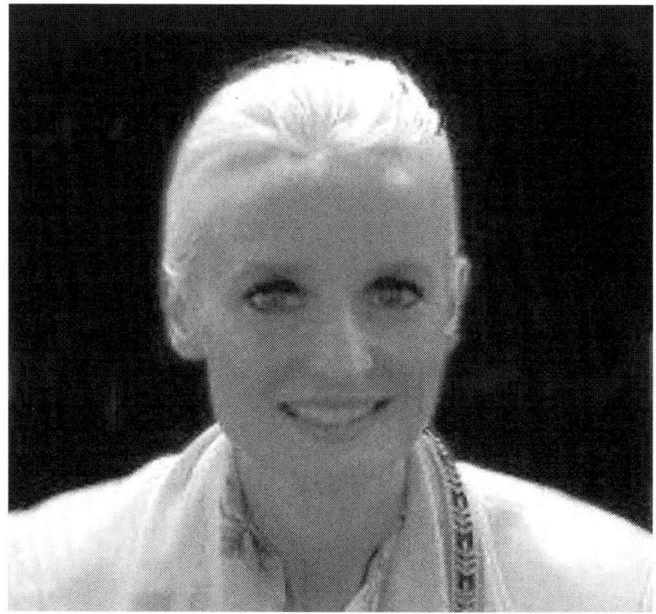

Bill: Janelle Ali-Dinar, PhD., Janelle is the Vice President of Rural Health for MyGenetx. She's also the Vice President of Strategy and Business Development for SelfCare for HealthCare and the COO of MedFirst Partners. Janelle is a national award-winning transformational leader, executive, and corporate strategist and communicator. Her demonstrated senior leadership as a CEO, COO, Senior Vice President, and Regional Executive spans the globe working with Fortune 500 companies and healthcare and hospital systems from Los Angeles to the Middle East, Europe, the Pacific Rim, all the way to rural America.

As a well-respected policy advocate at the state and federal levels, Janelle frequents Capitol Hill and serves on several state and national boards advancing rural, public, and minority health. Janelle has had great success teaching at, and facilitating within, rural and urban hospitals and clinics providing the principles and implementation formulas of transformational leadership. Janelle holds a doctorate in marketing communications, and recently graduated from a healthcare leadership institute at the University of Nebraska Medical Center College of Public Health.

She is currently involved in two ivy league leadership healthcare business programs and continues to provide leadership support in interim and long-term capacity hospitals and serves as Vice President of Rural Health at MyGenetx. Her goal in healthcare is to passionately and strategically build rural healthcare sustainability, whether it's keeping the doors of critical access hospitals open or recruiting physicians and specialists to providing leadership assistance to principals to new leadership teams as a guide, teacher, instructor, speaker, and mentor. Janelle, you are a busy person! Welcome to *Rural Health Leadership Radio™*.

Janelle: You are welcome! I appreciate that you would invite me to be a part of what is a great success as you launch this podcast. I'm very pleased to be one of your guests.

Bill: Janelle, you ae a very successful, driven, busy person! I don't know how you do it all. You are obviously passionate about leadership and healthcare, rural health in particular. Why did you choose healthcare as an occupation?

Janelle: Sometimes people will refer to me as another Energizer Bunny. It really kind of stems from the whole origin of passion.

Passion is really what is the drive and momentum and the energy to really do all of these things. For me, I am able to do this as not just the blessing of daily work, but really, it's an outlet of fun. With that creative and passionate energy, I never notice if I'm actually working or if I'm having fun. I found a way to unite the both of them. Looking at rural healthcare especially, there's plenty of opportunity to continually do that. Why did I choose healthcare as an occupation? I have to be transparent in saying that I did not originally choose healthcare. Healthcare is where I have been for fifteen-plus years now. A career in healthcare is a unique opportunity to get to see it from the lens of both the patient and from the lens of someone who works in it.

I do not provide clinical care, but I provide plenty of the operational and structural and strategic framework around that where I feel like I'm part of some of those clinical decisions. To me, healthcare is absolutely fascinating.

I actually started out in journalism, as a reporter extraordinaire. Then I began to work in management. From there, things really equated from the message and the deliverer of the message to the group of people to deliver and translate a message to. Suddenly, I then found myself working with physicians, which is really a great needed area to work with them. If you don't have physicians, it would not matter how many patients you have. I really cultivated a good working relationship around physicians.

Then it really evolved into part of what my training was in, which was strategy. From there, I kept the growing like most people do. I began climbing within the ranks of healthcare. Then those leadership job descriptions and titles then begin to grow as well. I've had an opportunity to be an EVP, to be a COO, to be a regional strategy director and executive, then to be a CEO as well.

Bill: I appreciate your passion for healthcare. You've worked around the globe, from Los Angeles to the Middle East, Europe and the Pacific Rim. Why have you focused on rural health?

Janelle: It stems from my own roots. I was born and raised a native of Nebraska. Really, the leadership lens and definition for me was really emulated having grown up on a farm and understanding where the roots are and how the soil is and how it seeds and the relationship of everything has to grow and work in harmony and collaboration. For me, even though I've had an opportunity to live across the world, to work across the world, and to live in large cities, it is always nice to develop those skillsets, develop that rich experience, and to be able to go back and give to a group, a community, a state, a region, where you can best emulate your skillsets, where you can best drive some results.

It's an opportunity to give back and to pay it forward, if you will. Having been from rural, I can't think of a better place to want to stimulate activity and stimulate results. As we know, there's a lot in jeopardy for rural healthcare, whether it's critical access hospitals or rural health clinics, or even the leadership workforce. Retention, recruitment, and what those job descriptions and what those communities will look like in the future. I think it's a wonderful opportunity to have developed the best and then to come back and give what I think is the best and that is in rural.

Bill: You mentioned leadership a lot in our conversation so far here. What's your definition of leadership?

Janelle: I think leadership is one of those things where you can have a nice working definition. But it is like mercury, it also is uncontainable. It needs to continue to grow and evolve as changes in dynamics and opportunities, both as adversity and as opportunities unfold themselves. I think structurally, or framework speaking, at the heart for me the definition of leadership is that it's authentic and deliberate pursuit, an investment of leaders listening, engaging, nurturing, activating, and optimizing the best of each person's strengths. Whether they are wanting to grow in their current role, wanting to expand into a different career pattern, just getting themselves started, or well-seasoned, maybe at a mid-career change, or those who are just constantly looking to learn themselves. The role of a good leader is to be able to mobilize and galvanize each of those areas that I talked about to really be able to develop strong leadership. When you lead, you're leading by example. I have always looked at doing to others as you would want them to do unto you.

I've had the opportunity to look back at some of the leaders that have shaped my own thoughts, my own decisions, and my own framework of leadership, for better or for worse, and to be able to extrapolate what I think are the best. If I could have built the most optimum definition of leadership, of what I wish I would have had, what I wish I would have received more of, and that which I would never want to utilize, what would that be? What I just delivered to you is really what my definition of leadership is. A lot of leadership is active listening and taking those pieces and putting that puzzle together. Then really developing some critical next steps. Leadership is never for self, it is always for others, for the good of the team, the good of the organization.

I think that's what's very powerful, that when we have an opportunity to shape, whether it's a small team, one other person, a department of five or ten other people, an expanded team of those that are reporting to you, or an entire organization of five hundred-plus, it's an opportunity to be actionable, to develop accountability mechanisms, and to really grow and invest and mentor and condition not only where the organization should be, but where your people are. They all have goals and objectives and dreams and job descriptions to fulfill. I believe there are always ways to create strategic opportunities to take what my definition of leadership is and really customize it according to what those needs are. That's the thing about leadership. It's that principle that it's always evolving and it's reviewing itself.

Bill: I appreciate that definition. I was taking some notes there. Some of the words I focused in on what you were saying were listening, engaging, mentoring, inspiring, sharing, all important components of leadership. Thank you for sharing your definition.

What would you say your top leadership strength is?

Janelle: I really have a few. It's kind of a run-on sentence, that when you look at it in terms of pillars. Inspiring is one of them, empowering is another. The result is the transformation. For me, it's to inspire and transform.

Bill: I appreciate your answer very much because what I like to do as a leadership scholar is compare someone's definition of leadership to what they try to do, as you said, lead by example. When someone talks about their leadership strengths, and they're the same things they talked about in their definition of leadership, that's excellent alignment. Thank you for sharing that.

You have worked with a lot of leaders in general, but particularly a lot of leaders in rural health. What leadership strength do you think is the most important for rural health leaders to be masters of?

Janelle: I have such great admiration for those who are working in leadership capacities in rural health. There is no set definition by virtue of proximity, zip code, or dynamics within resources. All the things within policy and workforce dynamics and within just where they are and where they work and what they're called to do in terms of being stretched in so many different ways and wearing so many hats is really the successful ability to adapt to change. I can think of no other industry that has had as many changes, especially since the Affordable Care Act was passed. A lot of the ACOs, the Accountable Care Act with ACOs and meaningful use and ICD 10 and all the different things that have happened as a result of its passage have really helped transform and add a lot of different deadlines and a lot of different projects to a lot of different areas of work. It's been an opportunity, but it's also been advanced timeframes and stresses and pressures. It prevents rural health areas of critical access health and rural health clinics to be able to survive let alone thrive. It's really been embedded upon them, but, in the meanwhile, they've had to adapt to a lot of change.

If you are someone who is highly structured, the rigidity of it sometimes lessens the ability to be able to adopt those necessary tweaks and changes that have to be made by virtue of policy, by virtue of changes in reimbursement, by virtue of changes within changing out an EMR system, or any of the different initiatives that critical access hospitals are called to participate in. If you can't adapt to that change, it makes it very difficult to lead your team through change knowing that there are some changes we can be in charge of but, for the most part, within healthcare, you can't. It's what you choose to do with those changes. I think if you can harness the power of change and you can use it to your advantage, you can use it as both a learning opportunity and a positive opportunity to help your team through this. It will also feel less burdensome for yourself as that leader. In change there should be transparency. There should be the availability and optimum capability to be able to share with your team so that they can help solve and evolve together. I think the power of change and being able to change successfully, to go with that flow, is really what's necessary for today.

Bill: Thank you, Janelle.

Speaking of change, can you share something unique that you've done, or you've observed other rural healthcare leaders do that worked?

Janelle: Absolutely. There have been a lot of success stories. Rural health leaders have a lot of job descriptions and job titles. Sometimes we forget that we are so much more than our job title. A job title just gives us a reference point, if you will, of how we're going to do our day-to-day work within a framework in context in terms of where my job begins. Is it a specialty area of expertise that might be handed off to another leader? What I've seen from the best successes is the mobilization of a campaign, a thought, a movement, a philosophy, if you will, that is called "We Are One." It doesn't change that a physician is a physician or that a PA is a PA or an APRN is an APRN, or if there's a C-Suite made up of the CEO and the CFO and clinical nursing. It is that everyone is going into a shared vision, mission, and purpose for why they are in an organization.

If you think about whether you are a community member or a patient or even someone who works within healthcare, those doors are open to the public. If you didn't have food services, if you didn't have maintenance, if you didn't have environmental services, if you didn't have a lot of the areas that people don't normally get a chance to interface with, if something went wrong, like the heating and the cooling system, or the hot water, or whatever the case might be, that could be the difference between keeping your doors open and not keeping them open. These core services are core pillars and why the doors are open. It's very important when you're thinking volumes of patients and where reimbursements are going, when you're thinking about operational cuts and budgeting, when you're thinking about all the things that are happening in the season of change within healthcare delivery, it's important that you bring all stakeholders to the table to be able to explain this is what's happening, this is what is needed. We would like to also tap into what some thoughts are within that. We would also like to listen to your concerns.

This “We Are One” campaign really puts everybody at the same. It doesn't change their job title. It doesn't change their responsibilities. It brings them all to the table to know and to understand, to listen, to exchange, and to plan for the future. When you've got that baseline of “We Are One” established, it's a lot easier than if there are policy changes and budget cuts needing to take place, or if there has been a change in how a 340B drug program has changed, or some other type of policy. While it may not be directly related to all of those, it is a puzzle piece that's very important for how the entire puzzle fits together.

"We Are One" as kind of a practice, if you will. It makes it much easier then to go on to those next layers. Tapping into each of those persons top four or five strengths and really finding ways to best tap into those. Sometimes it's taking someone who wouldn't otherwise have a speaking role, but recognizing that they do have a strength and a component necessary for leading teams and getting things to happen and being able to supercharge and ignite, if you will, all the steps that need to be done. It's a fabulous way of cross-referencing people's skill sets. It's a wonderful way to re-harness appreciation within that. Barrett has a wonderful program that's strength-based oriented. The Studer program where there's rounding with the patients. You should also round with your teammates. You should also self-round and take stock of where you are and your stress and how you're balancing everything. From a nursing standpoint, there's SelfCare for HealthCare.

There're lots of other programs that you can adapt as that second layer recognizing that that should be a continual flow of how information is shared and grown. I think the "We Are One" campaign has really demonstrated from the root some of those best success stories that I've seen. We've gone back a few years later and seen that it's still very evident. I feel the mantle has changed in leadership, but that next layer of leadership has really kind of taken that mantle. There's a sense of great pride in fulfilling the mission and vision of the organization demonstrated in these core principles of action.

Bill: Interesting. The "We Are One" campaign is a very interesting concept. Thank you for sharing that.

If we look at rural health leaders in general, what should leaders be thinking about for their facility and their respective teams in the rural environments?

Janelle: I think it's important they stay at the pulse of where policy is taking shape. In rural health, we've seen that there have been seventy-plus critical access hospitals that have closed over the last couple of years. We've seen another hundred and seventy-two on an immediate list. Another nearly seven hundred as a second layer of at-risk. I think you know what your risks are, that makes it easier to track what those pulse points need to be. From a rural standpoint for leadership, it's very important to be able to identify leaders that have a good grasp to understand what's at risk. I think it's also important to recognize that maybe not every critical access hospital will have a CFO. We're seeing a lot more CEOs acting as CFOs. We also see a lot of nurses stepping into the role of CEO, which I think is wonderful because they've grown up really understanding what their patient care needs are. That's another layer of additional strength.

It's going to be important strategically for healthcare leaders to position themselves where they need to be. Many of them want to stay independent. Rural has done a wonderful job within the leadership scope itself of collaborating and partnering with public health and partnering with other critical access hospitals. Providers themselves are thinking about ways they can demonstrate specialties and outreach clinics. Belonging to a clinically integrated network or an ACO is another option rural health leaders are considering where incentives are going allowing them to still provide quality care and have good benchmarks for patient outcome measurements and to create population health-driven communities where it's not just population of the community itself but really building on precision care.

CEOs today need to think about the following. They need to think about where critical access hospitals are going two and three years from now. We used to write strategic plans that were three years strong. Those are living documents and they're changing faster than ever. You can barely put your arms around a one-year strategic plan. They need to look at themselves operationally. Where do their margins need to be? Where is policy impacting them where they need to make some tweaks and changes? What would be a differentiator for them? They really need to develop a foothold within that marketplace. Look at what the competition is doing. Rural health are collaborators first, but they also do compete in a healthy way. Looking at some additional services, additional areas that they could be optimizing reimbursement. They should be listening to their patients, maybe take patient surveys, which is slightly different than patient satisfaction scores which are part of the HCAPS.

Rural health leaders really need to take stock in what their current patients need, what takes them out of town where they could otherwise be receiving care here? It's also important to be forward-thinking, to be looking at what CNF is offering in innovation models. If you can't compete in one area, where might you put some eggs in the basket, so to speak, to be able to apply for greater resources and develop some greater strengths? As we look at physician reimbursements, which are really going to drive things, we need to look at what best positions them. We know that when we look at national research, 70% of them are not meeting their benchmark threshold as it relates to meeting chronic care illness objectives, really getting to the root cost analysis of what's causing pain for their patients and how reimbursement is with that.

Rural health leaders need to look at the ACO's advance payment models. Of course, that falls under the range of MACRA, which is really where physicians are going to be receiving their reimbursements. We need to be thinking outside the lens.

As it relates to MACRA, we know that there has been some reprieve for rural. They may not have to participate in that, but now is not forever.

At the end of my sharing, it really is that CEOs, along with their core team, and even engaging their board members, they need to be actionably looking at what is the healthcare banner saying? What is CMS saying within the next two to three years that we need to be aware of so we can service and provide that ourselves. We can collaborate with others. We can position ourselves for that with a larger healthcare system under the wings of an ACL or a CRN. Or we can position our providers so that they're set up for success in the reimbursement model. I've said this before, I do believe that providers are your first patients. If you don't take care of your providers, it wouldn't matter how many patients you have.

The final item on this laundry list is to really look at where recruitment and rural workforce numbers and challenges are. We know that within ten years there will be a million-nurse shortage across the United States. In primary care, within the next ten to twenty years, it's a shortage of twenty to thirty thousand. When you look at those gigantic numbers, you can see within that framework of what do you need to be doing, what do you need to think about, so you don't have a shortage? That's thinking about looking at that next layer of people who are going to be emerging into the workforce, making rural and their site very attractive. It's thinking more organically that you might need to have a person wear more than one hat. You need to think more about a network of sorts.

The thing about being a CEO or a leader in rural health is that you're never charged with just one thing. It's the octopus with lots of tentacles. You're always changing and moving. You've got to get your tentacles, if you will, wrapped around all of these things. That's what's exciting.

Bill: Never a boring moment. That's for sure.

Janelle: Yes. That's right.

Bill: Janelle, you are a fountain of information. Thank you so much for sharing your thoughts, your observations, your experiences, your knowledge and your expertise in rural health.

Lisa Kilawee

Lisa Kilawee was our guest for this episode of *Rural Health Leadership Radio™*. At the time of our interview, Lisa was the President of the National Rural Health Association. During our conversation, Lisa to discussed her work and experience in rural healthcare and leadership. We also discussed the pioneering work she did with Avera and telemedicine in her career. Lisa touches on the work she has done as the president of the National Rural Health Association and the opportunities to become more engaged in rural health that are available through NRHA membership.

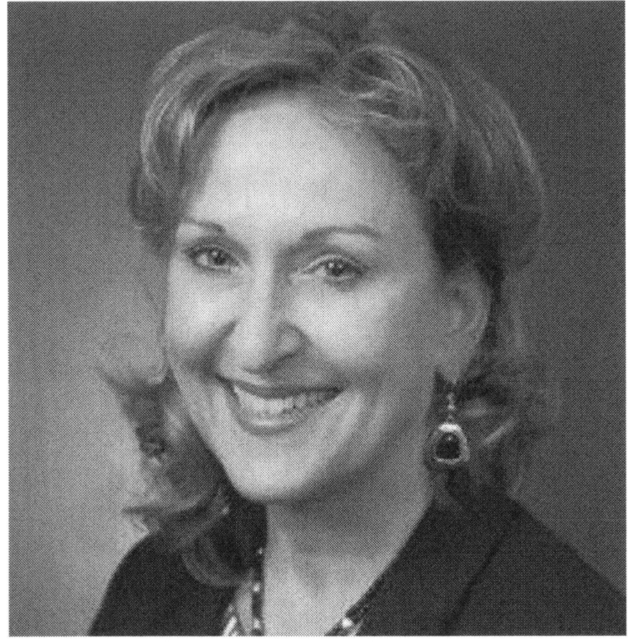

Bill: Lisa Kilawee is (at the time of the interview) the President of the National Rural Health Association. She is also a physician recruiter for Ascension Wisconsin, working in rural Stevens Point, Wisconsin. Lisa has a 30-year history of working with rural communities and a 25-year history of working in rural health and rural healthcare facilities. From the rest of what I'm about to tell you about Lisa, you'll realize she is a very busy person. She has a bachelor's and master's degree from the University of South Dakota and she's certified as a Diplomat with the American Society of Physician Recruiters. She's also an Ambassador for the Patient-Centered Outcomes Research Institute, and she's the current President of the National Rural Health Association. Her career has included working for the South Dakota State Office of Rural Health within the University of South Dakota Sanford School of Medicine, and for the Community Healthcare Association working with community healthcare centers, and as director of Rural Health Services for Avera Health in South Dakota for 12 years. Eighteen months ago, Lisa moved to the rural village of Amherst, Wisconsin with a population of 1,200 people, and works as a physician recruiter for Ministry Health Ascension Wisconsin.

You're obviously a very busy person who has dedicated 25 years to rural health. Why did you choose healthcare as an occupation to begin with?

Lisa: I was drawn to healthcare. Growing up, my family and my parents were always engaged in a lot of different social justice issues. When I went to school, I was drawn to community development and similar activities. That is how I ended up getting a Master's in Public Administration. My first job out of graduate school was working for a planning development district in all sorts of areas of community development and planning. I was always drawn from that end. I had the bug. I was also involved in telemedicine community planning. From there, I decided that my passion really was for healthcare.

Bill: That's great because we need people like you serving all of us in healthcare. Why rural health? There are a lot of different avenues you can take in healthcare, so why rural health?

Lisa: I was drawn to rural health because, right away, when I started working in healthcare, my father was diagnosed with a form of leukemia. Even though he lived in an urban community in South Dakota, South Dakota is still a very frontier state. This was 20 years ago, before the internet and everybody had Dr. Google. He was actually able to do some research and get involved in a clinical trial to get a bone marrow transplant in the next hospital-based university medical center, which was 4 hours from our home. That just really brought home the struggles that people from rural states have accessing all sorts of healthcare services throughout the continuum.

Bill: Yes, it can be very challenging. Transportation to and from is a huge issue.

One of the questions I ask everyone that comes on *Rural Health Leadership Radio™* is, what is your definition of leadership?

Lisa: My definition of leadership is someone that can take a grassroots approach and flip between whatever role you have, whether or not it's a formal leadership role, and you're able to energize whatever team you're working on to get things done. It is based on servant leadership.

Bill: I have to admit my prejudice. I am an advocate of servant leadership myself, so I appreciate you including that in your definition. Thank you.

You are the President of the National Rural Health Association, and you wear a lot of other hats, so you're definitely a rural health leader. What would you say is your top leadership strength?

Lisa: My top leadership strength is probably my grassroots approach. I really believe that everyone has a voice. If you watch me in a meeting or even at a party, you'll notice I'm talking to everybody. I'm talking to the caterer. I'm talking to the guy or the gal standing in the room by themselves. I think that everyone has a voice and the people whose voice may sometimes need to be heard the most are the people who are least likely to throw it out to you. I think that everyone in NRHA, and everyone who has worked with me, would agree that my grassroots approach to leadership is probably my top strength.

Bill: Listening to others and getting others to talk certainly can be a powerful tool for leaders to use. I appreciate that skill would be your top leadership strength.

In your variety of roles in rural health, you've not only been a leader yourself, but you've seen a variety of other rural health leaders. What strength do you think is most important for rural health leaders to be masters of?

Lisa: That's a really good question, Bill. I have had, as you said, the good fortune to work with a lot of rural health leaders. To borrow a phrase from a friend, a lot of rural health rock stars. One thing I know they all have is resiliency. One person in particular is Tim Size who started and still directs the Wisconsin Rural Health Cooperative. He didn't like the way things were going for rural communities in the job that he had previously, so he started his own initiative. You see that all throughout rural health. People standing up for what they believe in to make things better for the folks in rural communities.

Bill: Thank you. You just mentioned Tim Size and some of the things he did. Can you talk more about what he did?

Lisa: Tim created the Wisconsin Rural Health Cooperative. It's at least 20 years old. Tim believed that rural hospitals and clinics in rural Wisconsin did not really have a voice. And he was right, they didn't. At that time there were few facilities that belonged to larger systems and they were getting left out of the progress in healthcare that was being made. They were having a really hard time doing joint contracting and dealing with things like HMOs. His idea was that while maybe one organization couldn't afford these services and skilled professionals on their own, maybe if they collaborated with other or similar organizations, they could do that. So he helped them do that. He started by himself, and now he has a large staff, and they do some really great work.

Bill: Excellent. That's great utilization of resources to make things happen. Can you talk about any other unique things that either you, or others that you've worked with in rural health have done that has worked out well?

Lisa: I worked at Avera for 12 years, and it was one of the greatest things and greatest experiences that I will probably ever have. We made a decision as a family to relocate to Wisconsin, and the only thing that's missing here is Avera. I really miss the folks there. They do a lot of great work. Their senior leadership is really amazing. John Porter, their CEO, and Deanna Larson, the senior VP at eCARE and System Quality. I've been involved in telehealth for a very long time, since the late '80s, and it has really struggled. The efficacy is there and the evidence base is growing, but the payer structure and some of the minor technical issues need to be worked out. Especially regulatory and reimbursement issues.

Deanna Larson really had a lot of courage to not listen to nay-sayers. She continues to press forward and now she has a really robust telehealth service line that includes ePharmacy, eEmergency, eICU, and a number of services that are really transforming care. If you go to one of the facilities served by Avera eEmergency, you could be in Pukwana, South Dakota, or you could be in rural North Dakota, you would get the same care that you would get from board certified emergency physicians and trauma physicians that you would get in urban areas. She really had to put herself out there to do those things.

Bill: When you have the advantage of hindsight, when somebody else pioneers a purpose, a cause, or a service, it's easy to jump on the bandwagon afterwards. I can imagine as being part of the cutting edge of this, you're exactly right with reimbursement, we're still sorting all that stuff out. There were a lot of nay-sayers at that time, so that's a great example of leadership, of being a pioneer.

Bill: Sometimes we try to be pioneers though, and it doesn't work out too well. Have you ever, either yourself or witnessed another rural health leader, try something that didn't work?

Lisa: Never! Yes, yes of course. A lot of different examples; however, I'm not someone who's averse to risk, so I don't really think of them as failures. One of the earlier things when I first started working in rural health comes to mind. There was a huge physician shortage in rural and especially frontier states, which still exists today. Everyone was scrambling, trying to figure out how do we keep doctors in state, and the University of South Dakota Sanford School of Medicine came up with a really great number of strategies to try to retain and educate more physicians. One of the things we did, we rushed to put together a rural scholarship program to target physician's willing to commit early at the beginning of their medical school careers to practice in rural South Dakota. The tuition would be waived, and some other requirements would be waived. The idea was the physicians would commit to working in any underserved area.

Like a lot of things, as the program rules come out, it became clear as we worked through the details. A lot of the information we figured out at the end was with regard to how many underserved areas and federally designated underserved areas there were. We learned that often, there aren't clinics in those areas, so the options and communities available were limited. It might have worked out better if we had done education with that on the front end.

Bill: We don't like to have projects that we take under not go the way we planned, but sometimes we learn the most from those experiences. Since you're in the physician recruiting business, I'm sure you used that to your advantage moving forward from there. Thank you for sharing that.

With your experience with the variety of leaders you've seen and worked with, in your opinion, what do rural health leaders need to do differently?

Lisa: Looking at those rural health rock stars I have worked with, I think that most importantly, everyone needs to be open to change, and also resiliency. I look at a lot of different mentors that I've had. Going back to Avera, I think they're the only organization that has a Senior Vice President of Rural Health, and she's great. Her name is Rachael Sherard, my former boss. She really does a lot of great work and she was really resilient building the department, putting up with a lot of nay-sayers, really going through a lot, arguing with the work that she felt her department had to do. I would definitely say resiliency.

If you look at rural hospital administrators that are active in NRHA, they've really had to draw some lines in the sand with some of the organizations that they've been affiliated with. Sometimes that meant leaving organizations they were affiliated with because they no longer believed in their mission. I think resiliency is really important.

Bill: Very good! Resiliency! That is a great strength to have and the more resilient you can be in this changing environment, the more effective you can be as a leader.

One of the subjects that is a recurring theme when I talk to critical access hospital CEOs or rural hospital CEOs is the challenge of recruitment and retention of essential employees, providers in particular. You spoke to that a little earlier. I'm going to ask you a 2-pronged question here. What do you see as the advantages to being a rural healthcare provider versus working in the rural area, and what are the barriers to rural communities recruiting physicians for their communities and the opportunities there?

Lisa: The advantages are definitely there. It is a great lifestyle. When I look at our communities here in Wisconsin and the areas we serve and back to my work in

South Dakota with Avera, we have great communities that offer a lot of great aspects for quality of life. Basically, it’s the Norman Rockwell picture; homes with white picket fences and lots of recreation and lakes. It's all right out there by your backdoor. I talk with a lot of our rural physicians. They like being part of the community and being able to impact change. If there's something going on with their patients, if there's a mass layoff at a plant or something, they're acutely aware of those things, and they're there to help, to really make a difference. They are into helping the patient and the whole patient population. Not that you can't do that in urban, you certainly can, but it can be a lot harder to do. It seems like it's easier to touch lives in rural communities.

As far as the barriers, I'm a master troubleshooter so I really like to pick out some of those. You don't have that many. There's probably not a Macy's, so if that's important to you, or you might have to drive a few hours to get to Macy's. Sometimes, like I said, the work that Avera Health is doing with their eHealth service line is really helping, but before the advent of some of the current technology, the major complaint from rural physicians was that they felt isolated. They usually come from a residency training where they had mentors and all sorts colleagues at their fingertips, then all of a sudden, they're in a rural community. They may be the only physician and they have to make decisions on their own. The good news is that technology is addressing that barrier.

Bill: Having grown up in a rural community, there's a phenomenon that I refer to as the rural culture. If you're a physician you could be treating a family member one day, and then you're at the high school basketball game the next night. Everybody knows you. There's little to no anonymity. Some people struggle with that. Is that something that you've seen? If so, do you have any recommendations for dealing with that?

Lisa: Dr. Tom Dean is a rural physician in South Dakota. He was also a former NRHA President. I think he was practicing in a town of about 5,000 for most of his life. He talked about the trepidation he had about that. When he started, he actually took over the job that his father had had before him, so he had a lot of trepidation. He also knew that people in the community have a lot of respect for him. He thought it was funny. He was very private. He talks about how he was very private about giving out his phone number because he wanted to maintain his privacy. He was very careful about giving out his phone number. He said he had yet to receive a personal call from a patient at home. He thought, "Oh, I must be really good at protecting my phone number." Then he was down at the restaurant one night and it had been written on the wall. "In case of the doctor, call," and it had his phone number. But no one had ever intruded. I think most physicians that I talk to say that it isn't the problem that they thought that it might be.

Bill: Interesting. I had an acquaintance who was an orthopedic surgeon. He was recruited many years ago to a rural community on the Michigan-Canadian border. One weekend a year, this community allows snowmobiles to drive everywhere they want to drive during an annual festival. Normally, snowmobiles are not allowed on the roads; they have trails that they have to stay on. It just so happened, the weekend he and his wife went to visit the hospital and the community, it was the festival weekend. Snowmobiles were driving everywhere. His wife did not realize that that was an exception versus the norm. A day into the visit, she started crying and said to her husband, "I don't know if I can do this. I have to be able to drive a car." It was a simple misunderstanding about what the norm was there. Since then, he and his wife have raised their family in that same community. Sometimes there can be these perceived barriers that are not actual barriers.

You yourself, you just moved to Stevens Point, Wisconsin.

Lisa: Yes, I work in Stevens Point for Ascension Wisconsin. We live in the Village of Amherst, which is about 13 miles away, and it's a population of about 1,200. We have lived there for 18 months.

Bill: What have you learned about moving from an urban to a rural area?

Lisa: My number one lesson was that when you're actually experiencing something, it really hits home more so than knowing about it. For example, my daughter is in a rural high school. I really see the barrier that rural kids face, getting into health professions, training programs, even at a high school level, getting into those preliminary programs that are so essential to becoming part of a health profession program someday. It's all become real.

Bill: It has a whole new meaning for you, I'm sure.

Lisa: The tradeoffs are so worth it. We love it.

Bill: I think it's a great lifestyle, but I'm prejudiced.

As the President of the National Rural Health Association, what are the opportunities for anyone who may not belong to NRHA, or even if they do belong to NRHA, what can they do to get more involved? Basically, what can NRHA do for them?

Lisa: We're easy to find. We're on Facebook. We of course, like everyone else, have a website. People can certainly call me. We are always, always looking for new leaders. Right now, September 17th is the deadline, we're looking for our new officers and committee chairs. I'd be happy to help anyone out as far as how to get involved. At our annual meeting, we have conference sessions on informing people how to get involved. We have numerous standing and special project committees and we're always looking for volunteers.

Bill: I have two questions to close out our conversation, Lisa. What scares you the most about the future of rural health?

Lisa: What scares me the most is probably the reality that eventually tomorrow becomes today, so planning is really important. What excites me the most is that every day, we live in a really amazing time. Technology is advancing at a rapid rate. I remember the beginnings of telemedicine. Whoever thought that in reality people would be delivering and receiving healthcare over their phone? Very few people had phones when telemedicine first started. Mobile phones were in big bags in peoples' cars.

Bill: It is amazing.

Lisa: That really excites me, and also our rural health leaders excite me. As challenging as times are, especially right now, we have really amazing leaders. There is a lot of talk about the millennials, the younger generations and the new doctors. They look like teenagers to me. The fact is that these "kids" are all right. They have great values. They might work differently than people did in the past, but as far as mission and why they went into healthcare, it is incredible. I talk with so many great young doctors and they're all in. I think that is really exciting.

Bill: That's great! Thank you, Lisa!

If there's one thing our listeners should take away from our conversation today, what should that one thing be?

Lisa: Probably something one of my mentors, Tim Size, with the Wisconsin Rural Health Cooperative, once said, as well as another great person, Keith Kneeler: just because something didn't work in the past, doesn't mean it might not work in the future. In solving tough problems, we encourage people to have an open mind and consider all possibilities.

Bill: Thank you, Lisa, for sharing your thoughts and observations and experiences in rural health.

Teryl Eisinger

To celebrate National Rural Health Day, Teryl Eisinger, the Executive Director of the National Organization of State Offices, joined me for a conversation on *Rural Health Leadership Radio™*. We discussed how National Rural Health Day came about, the mission behind it, and the activities involved for the year. Over the course of our conversation, we also talked about many other rural health and leadership topics such as how rural healthcare is often associated with cutting edge technology and the national implications of rural hospital closures.

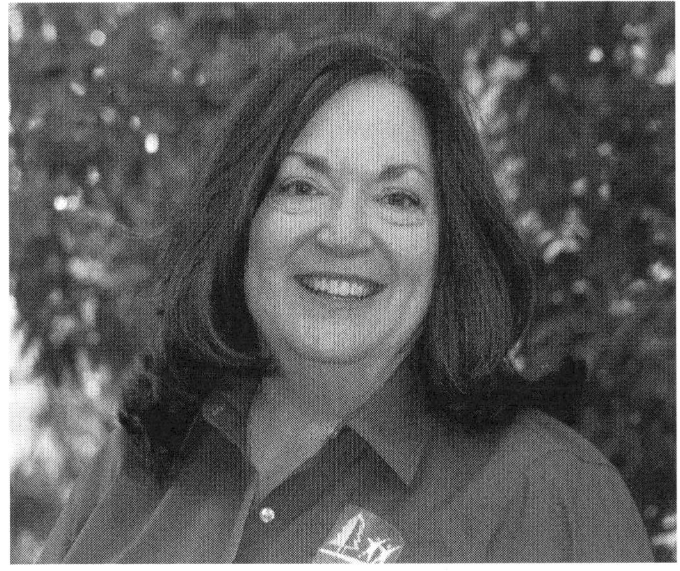

Bill: This conversation is a very special celebration of National Rural Health Day. To help us mark this special occasion is Teryl Eisinger, the Executive Director of the National Organization of State Offices, also known as NOSORH, which is a national non-profit membership organization that represents the fifty state offices of rural health around the nation. Created in 1995, NOSORH serves as an influential voice for rural health concerns, and promotes a healthy rural America through state and community leadership.

A long-time healthcare professional, Teryl has worked in rural health and health promotion for under-served populations for the past twenty years. Prior to taking the helm at NOSORH, Teryl was assistant director of the Nevada Office of Rural Health, and the Northeastern Nevada Area Health Education Center.

Throughout her career, Teryl has overseen a wide array of programming initiatives, including interdisciplinary training, state loan repayment, rural health outreach, abstinence education, and other federally funded programs. Teryl is a member of the National Rural Health Association, the Michigan Society of Association Executives, and the American Society of Association Executives.

She received her undergraduate degree in Allied Health Management from Northern Arizona University and holds a Master of Arts degree from the University of Nevada, Reno. She's taught communication, marketing, and business school courses at Great Basin College in Elko, Nevada.

Thank you, Teryl, for making time to be here. I do want to ask you a couple of questions before we get into National Rural Health Day. The first question, Teryl, is why did you chose healthcare as an occupation?

Teryl: It was always clear to me that a healthcare career is a great choice, especially if you're that kind of person who wants to help other people, and be part of something big. For me, back in those days, I thought that meant being a med tech or an administrator. Bill, I have to tell you, it only took me a few days as an intern at a small rural hospital for me to figure out that career path was not for me. I was very lucky that almost twenty-five years ago, about the start of the State Office of Rural Health Program I found my niche. I went to work for a state office of rural health and I have been there ever since.

Bill: Why rural health?

Teryl: I was living in a small town in Winnemucca, Nevada, and I was hired by the Nevada Office of Rural Health out of the University of Nevada School of Medicine as a community development coordinator. Back in those days, it was really very innovative for the Nevada Office of Rural Health to hire me. It was innovative what they called me too. I was a "telecommuter."

I wanted that. I really wanted to work from home and to be able to stay in a rural community. That work connected me with small towns. I was able to work with all kinds of community leaders, with EMS volunteers, and happy role model physicians who were out there doing hard work every day seeing patients. I could see how their work connected to what was happening on a national level, and I was hooked from then on.

Bill: You were a telecommuter before it was popular, so once again proving that rural health provides cutting edge innovation. We do celebrate National Rural Health Day this week, on November 17. How did Rural National Health Day come about?

Teryl: It was about seven years ago. I was with a member of my board and another colleague, and we were in Washington DC. The three of us were making an effort to visit large, well known health associations. We were trying to get them educated and excited about rural health.

Afterwards, we were standing on a street corner in DC. and Karen Madden, who is still the Director of the State Office of Rural Health for New York said, "Hey, we should have a National Rural Health Day." We really thought that would help educate associations and the public about the importance and key issues around rural health. From there, with the help of our members and all our partners, it just took off.

We want people to understand that small towns and small hospitals are working together with their state offices of rural health. They are doing great work to deal with the big challenges that rural people are facing as they seek healthier lives and better healthcare.

Bill: When I talk to people that work in healthcare in large urban centers, who've never worked in rural health, they often view rural health as just a smaller version of what they do. But it's nothing of the kind. It is much more complex. Was that part of the motivation for founding National Health Day, to point out those differences? I guess a better question would be; what was the motivation, in addition to what you've already shared with us?

Teryl: It really was about that. I think that the other thing we have tried to do is to turn it around. We often, in our advocate roles, really share widely the problems that exist in rural health. For us, it wasn't always apparent about the positive aspects of the kind of care that we've seen delivered in rural America. It’s a fact that you really can have high quality of care in rural. It's also a great place to live and work as a healthcare provider.

Yes, you're somewhat isolated. But you have an amazing opportunity to make a difference in people's lives every day while still addressing all those disparities and the differences that exist with the populations you deal with. There are also differences in reimbursement and other challenges too. We wanted to shout out about those differences and the positive nature of the care being delivered in small towns.

Bill: Is there anything else that we need to know or understand about National Rural Health Day?

Teryl: Yes! This year we're very excited about a lineup of great activities. We hope that people visit our website at NOSORH.org.

There will be a series of small, quick, visionary, thirty-minute sessions to educate people about dealing with the presidential decision and what it will mean for our country as we continue to try to transform our healthcare delivery system.

We'll be sharing lessons learned from helping communities to support their local hospitals, and we'll be asking them also to share a story about a community star. We'll be publishing a book on community stars. Most importantly, we'll be asking them to keep it going throughout the year, and to make the commitment to understanding rural America. I think it'll be a great day and just look forward to that blossoming and growing even more this year.

Bill: Excellent, thank you for sharing that information with us. Everyone in rural health knows that the number of rural hospitals closing each year is steadily increasing, and that one in three rural hospitals has been identified as being at risk of closing. How do rural hospital closings weaken our nation's health?

Teryl: It's a great question Bill, and I appreciate you bringing it up. This really is not a just a local problem. Certainly, the closure of a rural hospital is a real crisis in a rural community. I think that the most critical loss when a rural hospital closes, or is at risk for closing, it's truly the loss of a safety net.

In our country right now, we're tired of hearing about the fact that our health outcomes are worse, and we're spending more on healthcare dollars. We're working really hard to improve healthcare access for everyone, to improve the health of everyone. When a rural hospital closes, we're really losing a vital resource that will help us do just that.

The hospitals in many rural communities are the safety net provider and points of care for millions of veterans, senior citizens, farmers and ranchers, families and children, and for people who simply cannot afford healthcare. The loss of that safety net truly does weaken our nation's health.

Bill: The hospital closings make an impact on our rural population across the country too. Can you expand on that impact?

Teryl: I think one of the things that's the most difficult to watch as the community faces the rural hospital closure is the myriad of things that they're losing in those rural hospitals. In addition to being safety net providers, they are certainly focal points for emergency care. If a rural hospital closes, where are you going to take your child with a broken arm?

They're also really the brain trust of where the solutions about healthcare reside. When a rural hospital closes, that knowledge and expertise is really lost. There's not a focal point for, "Hey, how can we make this better?" I think even more importantly, for most people, is the employment factor. Rural hospitals are often one of the biggest employers in those small towns, and it has a big impact when people lose their jobs.

We know rural hospitals can be huge contributors to the economy. Our partners with the National Center for Rural Health Works measure this. I'm not going to quote their number exactly, but for every dollar spent on healthcare in a rural community, that will multiply back and make an impact in a rural community 1.2 to 1.5 times. That's a huge loss when a rural hospital closes. That doesn’t consider the impact on those folks that are working hard in economic development and trying to recruit new businesses into a small town.

Imagine having a business come check out your town and telling them there's no rural hospital. Imagine what it's like to be an emergency service provider, a volunteer on an EMT crew, and you only have a golden hour to get someone to the ER, and the next closest hospital is another hour down the road. What does that do to you? What does that do to your crew?

Other healthcare providers are impacted widely. When a physician is trying to keep a thriving practice going, and there's not a hospital in the town, how do they do that? Who does home health anchor with as they're providing services in the homes of people who are really frail? Home health agencies need that support. Just look at the community agencies at large, the schools and the other human services providers. Everyone from the police to the local WIC office feel it when a hospital closes. It's a tragic loss. We have to do the best that we can to help rural people find the care they need, especially when they're dealing with that issue.

Bill: The total impact is incredible. When you tell those who live in urban areas about this, everyone gets the fact that if a rural hospital closes, people are going to have to travel for healthcare. I'm surprised at how many people outside of rural health don't realize that total impact of a rural hospital closure.

Thank you for sharing this information.

Teryl, in your opinion, what do rural health leaders need to be doing differently? What do they need to be doing to address some of the challenges we've been talking about?

Teryl: We've just finished a tool kit to help our members help rural leaders address that. Closure certainly is tragic for a community, but it can also be a rallying cry for communities to work with their neighboring towns, to get creative and think about what people really need. It forces them to undergo some decision-making processes to plan for what actually is needed in terms of day to day services. It also provides the opportunity to make connections with other providers, maybe in urban areas, maybe with the next closest small town.

There is some real promise in the innovative work that's happening. We've watched our South Carolina Office of Rural Health do things like transformation projects and loan pools. There's a lot of meaningful collaboration that can make things better for rural communities if they have a vulnerable hospital, or even if they don't. That innovation is really happening all around the country.

Bill: Yes, it is. We see it every day, but it's always good to hear about it.

Can you talk about something unique that you've observed a rural health leader implement in their organization that had a positive impact?

Teryl: Yes! That's what keeps me coming to work every day! I'm excited about so many things that I see. Last week I was at a meeting at the Federal Office of Rural Health Policy. They brought together their community outreach grantees. There was a story shared from northern Maine, about medical supplies being delivered by a drone. I found that very exciting! One thing that I've watched over the years is the adoption of this technology and the transition of care. This transformation is truly happening around the country.

I think what's exciting to me is that it's really rolling out in the everyday operations of hospitals and rural health clinics. We're watching folks like the Michigan Center for Rural Health pull together collaborative groups of a couple of accountable care organizations. They're able to do this work based on work that they've done before, getting rural hospitals to participate in quality networking activities, and other ways to benchmark with each other. That builds and makes a position so they can see that they can build from there and be more creative.

It's so fascinating to look at the quality of care that is really improving because directors of nursing, and directors of quality improvement, and administrators are all in it together. And they love sharing their stories. The outcomes are there. We are seeing in study after study that rural hospitals are delivering a quality of care within their scope of work that is equal or better to many of their urban counterparts. I'm very excited to see that happening.

Bill: Yes, that is great news!

Sometimes we learn the most from trying things that don't necessarily work the way that we had hoped. Can you talk about something that you've seen a rural health leader try that didn't necessarily work out the way they had hoped?

Teryl: It's a collection of work around telehealth. I don't know about you, Bill, but I'm a baby boomer; I grew up watching the Jetson's. To me, it should not be rocket science that we can make these connections for rural people through telehealth. It baffles me why, when patients will accept that kind of care, when they understand what it's saving, that we cannot get out of the way of the smart physicians and the regulators to help these kinds of services be reimbursed. This work has been possible for many, many years, and it's still an uphill battle. That really needs to change, and it surprises me every day when I hear about another obstacle. I think we're making some strides though.

Bill: Yes. Definitely making strides, but I understand what you're saying. What do you think rural health leaders need to do differently?

Teryl: What I believe that rural health leaders need to do, is to be fully informed, and to engage and have a way to filter information that makes it meaningful for them to do that. It's really hard to keep up. What you are doing with your stories, I think, is highly impactful.

We're launching a pledge this year as part of National Rural Health Day, and we're asking that rural health leaders continue to do things differently by making a commitment to educate, to communicate what their needs are and the needs of others. To innovate, and to keep on collaborating. I really think that those four things are the key to what all rural health leaders need to do, no matter what position they're in.

Bill: Excellent, I like those. What is the future of rural healthcare?

Teryl: I'll just give you Teryl's version: I like to imagine and see a possibility for a future, where primary care providers and hospitals in rural communities are really getting the recognition for the good care they provide to people, right where they live. I would to imagine and see a possibility for the future that these providers and their patients are meaningfully networked to other higher levels of care that can easily provide services for them.

Also, that they're grounded by a true local commitment to coordinating care, to using data locally to make good decisions, and to taking care of patients right where they are. I really believe that that's a possibility, especially in rural America. The potential is there, we just have to get out of their way.

Bill: What scares you the most about the future of rural health, Teryl?

Teryl: I guess, really, that we won't realize that vision. When you take a look at what's happening with increasing costs of premiums across rural America, the lack of choices for those providers and the types of providers seem to be shrinking. I think that at the root cause of a lot of that is truly a lack of understanding rural healthcare, about the payer mix in rural America and the value of primary care services.

There might be a bit of a prevailing mindset among some regulators or policy makers that rural people, senior citizens, veterans, children, and families, don't deserve the same kind of care, just because of where they choose to live. National Rural Health Day is about changing that perception.

Bill: I asked you what scares you the most, what excites you the most about the future of rural health?

Teryl: I'm so excited about the work of our state offices of rural health and the facilities that they work with and the partnerships that they push along, sometimes just even in the background. They are making a real difference for rural people. I love seeing the projects when we're integrating primary care with behavioral health or oral health, or we're getting a behavioral health specialist into a primary care setting. Or the other way, where people kind of have that real place where they know they can be taken care of.

I'm very excited to see the good work that's being done to promote new models for healthcare. The shortage of doctors isn't going to change, I don't think, any time in the near future. If we can learn from the lessons, from people who are doing projects around community paramedicine, and really utilize community health workers and therapists, tap into and pay for the promise of that technology, and the drones, and telehealth, and all of that, that makes it worth showing up to work every single day.

Bill: That is exciting. What do you hope National Rural Health Day will accomplish this year?

Teryl: As I said, we really want people to know that rural America is a great place to live and work. It's a place where you can make a difference in people's lives. We want people to go out and find out what's happening in their community around rural health.

Bill: That's a great goal to accomplish. Is there anything else that you would like to say about National Rural Health Day, before I ask you my last question for the day?

Teryl: Just how to share the message. Use the #powerofrural on Twitter and in your social media. Share what you love about rural

America on November the 17th. Let us know how we can help further your message of what you're trying to do with your good work.

Bill: Thank you. We've talked about a lot of different things here: advances in rural health, concerns, what's working, and what's not working. If there's only one thing that people take away from our conversation, what would you like that one thing to be?

Teryl: Bill, it's not going to be one thing, but I can wrap it up with our National Rural Health Day pledge. That is that we want people to pledge to educate, communicate, innovate, and collaborate. That's the key to all of this good work that we're all trying to do.

Bill: Excellent, great summary. Thank you, Teryl, for having this conversation and sharing the significance of National Rural Health Day, as well as sharing your thoughts, observations and experiences in rural health.

Gary Lucas

Gary Lucas is Vice President of Education Operations at the Association for Rural Health Professional Coding. This conversation provides an in-depth look at billing and reimbursements in the rural healthcare industry. Gary explains what he believes to be the three most important things and the three biggest mistakes in these areas and provides examples of how improvements could be made to make not only these areas work better, but the healthcare system as a whole.

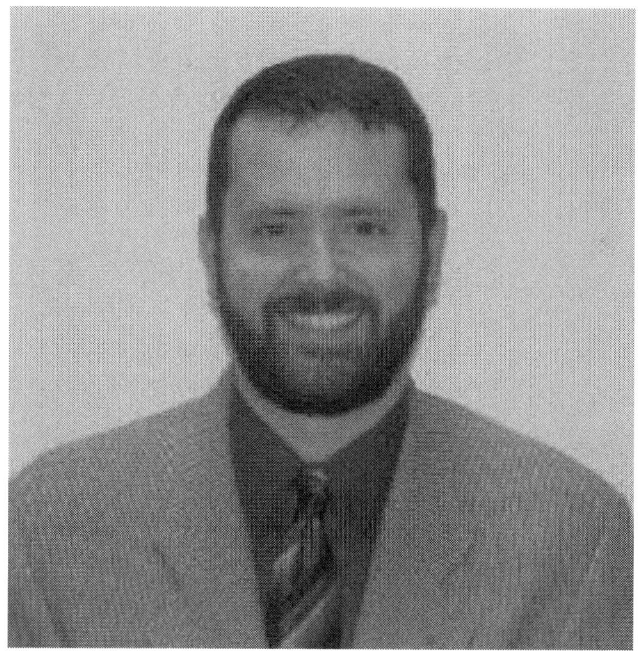

Bill: Gary Lucas is the Vice President of Education Operations at the Association for Rural Health Professional Coding. Gary currently serves as both Senior Faculty and Vice President of Education Operations for the Association for Rural Healthcare Professional Coding while serving the state and federally funded medical community. Gary has a particular focus on helping rural health federally qualified public and school-based health centers to manage the integration of clinical documentation regulations into their healthcare organization's business operations, such as professional coding, medical billing, and compliance auditing by educating staff who can carry out a plan to unify its people, its processes, and it's supporting technologies.

Gary's primary focus is to create educational collaborations with state rural health primary care and hospital associations who seek to help the careers of their members and improve the financial success of their member medical facilities through ongoing education.

He earned his Masters of Science degree in health informatics from the University of Illinois, Chicago, in March of 2014, preceded by a degree in Business

Administration from the University of Georgia's Terry College of Business in 1994.

Gary enjoys attending sporting events, finding hole in the wall restaurants, playing and watching live music and making his two sons laugh. Welcome, Gary!

Gary: Thank you, Bill, it's a pleasure.

Bill: Gary, why did you choose to focus on rural healthcare in your occupation?

Gary: Well, it's been an interesting track. My journey in this industry began back in 1994, and throughout the course of my 22 years in this industry, I've had the opportunity to travel and teach about 1,600 full day courses on these topics in over 46 states. We focused on larger towns at first. After the first 18 years, a colleague of mine and a former associate had really begun focusing on rural health when he noticed there were not adequate resources or educational resources focused on the unique needs of rural health. At the time, I looked back and realized when I was on an airplane that I was flying to Chicago, that I was flying over a heck of a lot of people that would never be able to make it up to Chicago to get this type of support.

Gary: It really reinforced for me the need for companies such as ours to provide that level of support because rural health has a lot of unique challenges, not only with the scarcity of resources and difficulty in retaining providers, but in physically getting themselves to a class to handle the ongoing education.

My mother was in healthcare, and she's from rural Illinois. Her experience had an impact on me. I knew first hand that these are people that often don't have the same career opportunities as are in-large cities, and there are a lot of folks that we want to help get a career in healthcare and not just have a job.

The more I started to think about it, the health of a rural health facility, the financial health I should say of a rural health facility, does impact the overall economy. I recently heard about a rural hospital in Alabama that closed along with the two clinics in the same area. There was a factory that was looking to relocate to that area, but decided they had to go elsewhere because there wasn't access to quality care. Whether it's from the individual needing the support to have a 20, 30-year career in healthcare or to the facility that is not able to send its people to get traditional education, it's just a slam dunk when you realize if all you're doing is going to the major cities, you're leaving a lot of people out.

Bill: That is very important. Thank you, Gary, for sharing that perspective. You definitely provide leadership in healthcare. What's your definition of leadership, Gary?

Gary: I had a chance to think about this, because I know this is an area that you focus on.

I thought about how to go about defining leadership and a quote popped up in my head. I think it's unattributed, I'm not sure who said it, but it says, "To a person who knows not to where they sail, every wind is favorable." What I've seen in our particular area is the ability to clearly define achievable goals and to forcibly work a plan with people who are empowered to make decisions toward that plan and really to not sacrifice anything getting closer to that goal is true leadership. Some facilities that I've had the opportunity to work with and other anecdotes that I hear from colleagues in the industry and certainly in some cases, survival equals success. The doors are open, we're used to running small margins; we're used to not being able to expand our facilities in a manner as traditional facilities do. Some of the items in my particular area of expertise merge leadership and finance.

The goals that we set forth in our field really are pretty clear.

Number one, are you able to document every service that's provided? That's a challenge, but we should be able to develop systems that require our providers to document everything that's done. However, there have been leadership challenges in the field because some EHR companies and some software companies make some promises that don't necessarily hold true in the real world. It's difficult to adjust for some of those unanticipated consequences of some of these decisions.

You go back to manual work arounds or the way it was done in the past. Or you can provide leadership by confirming with physicians that they have an obligation to document their care. It’s not just for the facility, but for the patient's benefit. We feel that that's something that shouldn't be sacrificed. We hear from leaders outside of class that yes, I know that's an admiral goal, but if I tell my providers to do that, they're going to leave. I recognize the difficulty, and working with providers and adding more coding and documentation responsibilities is proven to be challenging.

Gary: Sticking with clear goals, staying steadfast in pursuit of those goals, and really trying not to ever sacrifice on survival is essential. Focusing on what you need to do to thrive and the ability to define clear goals will provide everybody, with a shared direction. The ability to make those shared goals clear and attainable provides everybody with a foundation they can use to look back on.

Document 100% of what you do. Capture 100% of what you've done in terms of the procedures, services and diagnoses. Make sure that you're receiving every bit of revenue you're entitled to but not one more dollar than is allowed. That is something that would be hard-pressed to counter. It would be hard to convince me that we shouldn't document everything we do, that we shouldn't be able to extract all of the data out and generate revenue. Clearly defined goals are essential.

Bill: That's good. I love your definition. Anytime you use a sailing analogy I'm all in.

You have already spoken to my next question a little bit, but let me ask, what are the top three things that a rural hospital CEO needs to know about billing and/or reimbursement?

Gary: Excellent. I'm going to come about this from a couple different perspectives, things that I'm seeing that are being done well and other areas where I hope to continue to be able to help make some changes. Number one is in the past, those individuals that have been given the responsibility as a coder or as a biller or sometimes both. These individuals have traditionally worked their way up to that position. They tend to start working at the front desk of a facility, which doesn’t really require extensive training. You do need good public service skills and customer service skills for that position. Over time, some of their responsibilities change; however, they're not given recognition as being a high-level professional that deserves to have a focused and open communication line with the providers.

In the past, those associated with coding and billing have had great difficulty opening up lines of communication with providers to the point that if I grabbed a coding book and started walking down the hall and see a provider and I need to ask a question, the moment they see me with that coding book in my hand, they tend to run the other way. Because these individuals work their way into these positions without traditional education, my sense is that a lot of providers, through no fault of their own, are not seeing these people as the only people in the facility that are being given the ability to turn clinical documentation into revenue. You have a lot of people having to make very important billing decisions without the ability to communicate with providers on a regular or routine basis. A lot of times when they go to a manager or supervisor regarding these issues, they're often told, "Look, do what you need do to get the client paid, and let's not bother the providers." Number one is open up a clear, routine, and effective line of communication between those who create clinical documentation and those that turn that documentation into revenue.

That feeds into my second area, which is to provide education and training for these individuals and for the providers. In my 22 years of teaching, I've been responsible for learning 23 different versions of the CPT manual. Of course, we just underwent the large change from the ICD-9 to the ICD-10, and in reality, one of the reasons this entire company was formed is a colleague of mine was teaching in a state down south and the person came up after class with a question. He said, "Let me take a peek at your coding manual, and I'll show you where the answer is," and their coding manual was four years old.

Gary: This is an area of healthcare that constantly changes. There are continual documentation and coding updates.

Medicare and Medicaid are constantly making adjustments to payment policies. That requires those individuals to go back and identify to the providers what those changes may be. If you have education at the forefront, then you have already built a process by which those updates can be gathered, implemented and monitored and changed as necessary. The fact is, we have been amazed at finding out how difficult it is for some facilities to just get their coders and billers the proper coding manuals every year. It is somewhat amazing when you're looking at about a $200 investment with the one individual that's responsible for bringing in tens or hundreds of thousands of dollars a year.

Again, number one is creating effective communications between the clinical providers and those on the coding and billing side.

Number two, is documenting and planning for a commitment for an ongoing education and training plan that mixes in-person learning, distance learning and e-learning. It should also create touch points throughout the month or quarter, where everybody can get together and really discuss these as opposed to a lot of the training that we see that really happens in stove pipes. The clinical provider is going to get their training from one area, the coders get it from another area, and everybody tends to follow some of those guidelines they like. There's really not a mixing of those two items.

Number three is the importance of retaining these individuals. We often focus on the importance of retaining providers, but I would argue that it is just as important for their retention. It's not often in this field that you have a pool of people in your community with the aptitude and trust to hand over the reins of putting the facility's tax ID number on the claim form and asking Medicaid for state tax money and asking Medicare for federal tax money. Credentialing is important. Providing these people not only with an important job and the support they need is important, and so is recognition. There are various certifications and credentialing options out there that can give these people a sense of pride. By giving these individuals the opportunity to see themselves and others as a high-level professional is an area where you're going to be able to retain them.

Gary: These people can see that survival doesn't always equal success. When you have an education and a training plan that utilizes internal and external resources you enhance success. You know that you're not just doing it the way you were taught. You may have a person who learned from the person who learned from the original person ten years ago, and that is not a winning formula. Those all tie together, and that starts at the top with a commitment from leadership.

The last item I will ad is technology. Technology continues to run its way into the daily lives of providers and coders and billers. This presents a challenge because you're dealing with a lot of disparate systems that don't often talk to each other. Sometimes the folks that are in my area, the coders and the billers and the EHR folks, aren't involved in active discussions about upgrades or feature sets or how things should be organized when they're the ones that are actually touching it on a day-to-day basis. Hopefully, these ideas help organize some of the thoughts that the C-Suite folks need to do.

Bill: Yes. Thank you, Gary.

I like to focus on our successes, Gary, but sometimes we learn the most from mistakes we've made. What would you say are the top three mistakes that you see rural hospitals make related to coding and billing?

Gary: That is such an excellent question. I think there's too much of a reliance on technology to do a job. Whether it's extracting the codes from the documentation or if it's simply sending that list of codes through a practice management system to help organize and identify the bill, there are a lot of problems there. For example, inside an electronic health record, an EHR often advertises that it can give your providers a recommend action, what's called an evaluation and management code. These are your office visit codes or your hospital visit codes that are reported, or coded I should say, based upon the documentation of history and the documentation of exam. This is what the AMA has identified since 1992 as medical decision making.

There is too much of a reliance on a system as opposed to an educated individual. Without getting too much into the weeds, an electronic health record has the ability to calculate the level of history based on the CPT definitions. In 1995 and 1997 and in several other years, Medicare really expanded upon and clarified those definitions. The way that most EHRs are set up can help you figure out your level of history because of the way the EHRs are organized.

When you move to a level of exam, there are two different sets of guidelines that Medicare allows us to use. Generically, they are called the 1995 and the 1997 exam guidelines, and Medicare to this date has not mandated that we use one or the other. Because of that, I hesitate in trusting an electronic health record in understanding whether I should use one or the other. Believe it or not, it can change with different patients and it can change with different payers.

When you get down to that area of medical decision making, there's no EHR that can put itself in the mind of the provider to help understand the level of risk associated with that patient's co-morbidity. There is a thought process behind analyzing the amount and complexity of diagnostic data a provider uses to determine diagnosis and management options. We've had several providers come say, "Well look, I always just pick the recommended code popping up in my EHR," and when we show them the potential for issues, it really raised a lot of eyebrows. For example, in rural health, traditionally there is one bulk or one group payment rate with Medicaid. No matter what they do for the most part, they get one all-inclusive rate for everything that's done.

To move onto my second common billing mistake, which dove tails with the first, is a lack of understanding in the industry overall. Rural health providers often say, "Hey, what does it matter what level of service I report when Medicare is going to pay me the same dollar amount?" Well, there's a big issue there because some changes we went through in the industry as of April 1st, 2016. For example, the way the patient's charges, the way the patient's code insurances are created is based on my charge for the service, not Medicare's payment.

If I'm coding consistently level three visits when I'm actually performing level four visits, there are significant opportunities for revenue. If the patient doesn't have the ability to pay, we move to a sliding fee scale and other financial options. The impact of this mistake is going to result in additional revenue being lost. Not only from patient co-insurance amounts, but what about that 20% to 30% of those patients with commercial insurance?

The third common mistake is to report services to commercial payers as if it is the same billing guidelines that Medicare requires. The short version is commercial insurance companies sometimes pay for things that Medicare won't. If we're dropping that off the claim because, "Hey, I'm the coder and biller, and I've been told just turn this documentation into a check," but if that's a commercial carrier and I haven't reported the correct dosage units of inject-able drugs, that can be tens or hundreds of dollars just on one claim. That goes back to, "Medicare was going to pay me the same." But be it Blue Shield or Aetna or Traveler's or whoever, that could have been another hundred dollars in viable, justifiable appropriate revenues.

Number one, over-reliance on technology. Number two, not focusing on the thing that happens every day and that is your evaluation of management coding and relying on software. Third, not recognizing the negotiating power with rural health clinics when it comes to contracting. The benefit of a lot of hospital systems purchasing rural health clinics, is they do have and they should be able to exert that negotiating power based on the broad scope of patients that they're able to take care of geographically. With the advent of the essential community provider, commercial insurance companies are obligated to make a genuine effort to include facilities like rural health clinics in each and every one of their commercial insurance products.

There are more detailed nuances to it, but we really hope that the rural health CEO confirms how and if they can participate in the essential community provider area. At that point, you're going to have the opportunity to generate revenue that you're not used to getting from Medicare. In summation, documentation doesn't change based on the patient type. We're going to provide the same care to every patient no matter what insurance they have. Therefore, the coding doesn't change based on payer type. The codes are simply a reflection of what's in the medical records documentation, and we want people to code each and every item that was done, each and every diagnosis on why it was done, whether it's separately reimbursable or not. This way you're going to be able to pull a lot of data out that has nothing to do with revenue that can tell you what you're actually doing.

As we move towards outcome-based reimbursement, doing pay for performance. Documentation doesn't change, coding doesn't change, but when it comes to billing, Medicare does lead the way. But Medicaid does things differently, and each commercial plan out there might require you to adjust that bill based on their unique rules. While the documentation coding never changed, you better believe that those bills need to look different. A lot of software being used by rural health clinics prepares the claim as though it were a Medicare fee for service claim, not a rural health clinic claim. There's an opportunity for a lot of revenue, but you could be getting paid for things that you shouldn't be billing out.

Bill: The more I listen to you, Gary, the more I realize how education in this area is vitally important to the health and financial well-being of the organization.

How important do you see the value of earning credentials for non-providers in rural health?

Gary: Traditionally, they have not had the opportunity to do that. There are some wonderful organizations out there that offer well-recognized coding credentials. We happen to offer our own credential that is unique to Rural Health. We do not replace AAPC and/or HEMA credentials, but rather hone in on what the rural healthcare market needs are. One of the things lacking traditionally in some of the more well-known credentials is they don't cover billing. While the coding piece is absolutely important, a lot of people in rural facilities that go to get these certifications have to learn and spend a lot of money to learn cover to cover, all of the different manuals. In actuality, they receive credentials they're never going to use in a rural health. Our philosophy is that you need to learn the coding piece of and while focusing on what you do on a daily basis

Our credentials, and others, should be used together so that people's business cards are as wide and long as a piece of paper, because those are credentials they can take with them if they move out of rural. It's also useful if a larger facility purchases a clinic. It shows that they have gone that extra mile. One of the great things about credentialing is that once you earn the credentials, you have them forever. Of course, you have to earn continuing education units. Those continuing education units should be tailored on a traditional staple of services done in a rural health center. To leave the billing piece out of it is not ideal. One comment we often hear is, "So wonderful, you taught me how to code, that's great. Now I need to take these eight codes and figure out which three I'm going to get paid for." Again, that's different from Medicare than it is Medicaid.

The value is to show our commitment to helping them in their career, and then the financial benefits come to the facility through a higher level of professional service. We want to ensure that those trained professionals capture everything being done and everything being done is getting paid for. It's the right thing to do.

The traditional salaries for non-credentialed people compared to credentialed people are significantly different because the impact of that credentialed individual is much higher. Lastly, you want to show you have a board-certified provider, and you have a certified biller and coder.

If I had the choice between somebody that's been in the industry eighteen years without a certification and somebody that's been in the industry for two years, but has a certification, I need to give that second person a shot because just because you knew how to do it eighteen years ago, doesn't mean you know what you are doing today. I'm not disparaging those that have been in the industry a long time, but their credentialing and ability to maintain that on an annual basis is essential. You have that added level of security that if something goes wrong, you can prevent this from happening. The CEOs that are listening want to be able to prevent this. You don't have to do anything wrong to get sued. You may not have done anything wrong to get audited by an insurance company.

If they start looking at things in the fraud versus abuse area. Having credentialed individuals that perform routine internal audits of documentation and coding and billing processes can help prevent trouble. Even if they find a mistake, it is unlikely that a third party doing the external audit is going to be able to prove fraud. Fraud typically indicates that there was an intent to mislead the insurance company. Whereas it could be, the legal term for abuse I think the legal term is called "oops." You know, "Oops. Okay, we did that one wrong," but you can't prove intent. Yes, that's there, but in terms of lessening fines and lessening exposure, a credentialed individual is going to be able to look into the issue, extract the source material, identify what's really happened in the past, and hopefully before those audits happen, with that clear and effective communication to both leadership and providers, make changes to prevent exposing the organization to some of those audits.

Bill: Gary, we've talked a lot about a lot of different topics here, even though it's all on billing and coding. It obviously can become a rather complicated discussion, but you break it down into simple terms.

If our listeners only take away one thing from our conversation today, what's the one thing you would want them to take away?

Gary: Retire? No! I'm kidding! That was terrible! In all seriousness, it goes back to my central theme. I have spent 22 years trying to make this field be recognized as being vital to the success of not only one person's career, not only to the health of that facility, but also vital to helping patients so they have a clear understanding of what's happening. We don't open our offices to run a 340-B program. We don't open our offices to submit medical claims. We open our offices to provide medical care to those that need it. If we're not placing a laser-focus in terms of support, education, and access, if we're not putting a laser-focus on the center of that revenue cycle, after all, we open the doors to provide care and to document it and to get paid for it, then I just want to see that area. That dove tails with getting providers engaged in the process.

I can't tell you how many people we provide a wonderful education. Afterwards, they come up and say,

"Everything was great; thank you for the information, but you can tell me this all-day long. Until my providers hear it, it's not going to matter." Getting providers in these classes, recognizing that it's hard to take a day or two away out of the office to attend these classes. That will show providers that these are not just people that were working the front desk six months ago and are now doing coding without a formalized degree. These are the people that have a job that requires high-level critical analysis skills that don't determine the health of a patient but really are central to the health of the facilities and their ability to stay open next year while all the time, undergoing a lot of change.

Bill: Thank you, Gary, for carving out time to share your thoughts and your expertise in the billing and coding world of rural health.

Dr. Mike Keegan

Dr. Mike Keegan is an infectious disease specialist with more than 25 years of experience in the medical field. During our conversation, we discussed rural health and leadership. As an infectious disease specialist, Dr. Keegan has dedicated much of his career to decreasing the dependency on broad spectrum antibiotics. Much of our conversation focuses on the antibiotic stewardship program Dr. Keegan helped create, which helps promote this goal, as well the benefits of antibiotic stewardship from several angles including health and economic benefits.

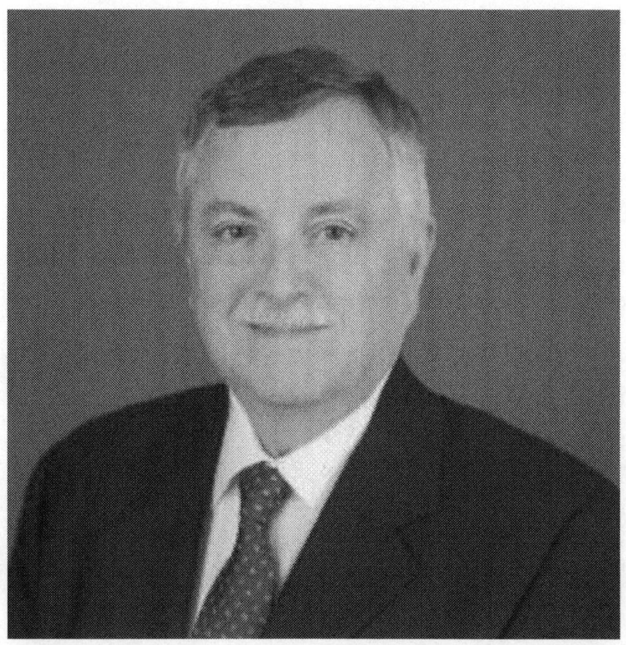

Bill: Dr. Mike Keegan is the Principle Healthcare Consultant with Pershing, Yoakley, and Associates. He is an infectious disease specialist with more than 25 years of experience in the medical field, and he serves as his firm's antibiotics stewardship program service line leader. Throughout his career of practicing medicine, Dr. Keegan has taken an active role in improving the quality of healthcare and patient outcomes by serving in numerous medical director and hospital executive leadership positions. Dr. Keegan has taken a special interest in solving the negative impact of the over-reliance of broad spectrum antibiotics. He has designed and implemented numerous successful antibiotics stewardship programs that have shown a decrease in the incidents of drug resistant bacteria.

Some of the titles Dr. Keegan has held during his career include Medical Director of Antibiotic Stewardship, Medical Director of Infection Control and Chief Medical Officer at healthcare facilities and systems in South Dakota. He founded a healthcare consulting firm centered around the provision of antibiotic stewardship programs for hospitals and communities across the country and is a consultant to the South Dakota Department of Health regarding antibiotic stewardship.

Dr. Keegan has also served as a Clinical Associate Professor at the University of South Dakota School of Medicine and has authored multiple articles and publications related to antibiotic stewardship and other infectious disease related topics.

Dr. Keegan, I'm truly honored to talk with you.

What is your definition of leadership?

Mike: Leadership in the information age is best defined by servant leadership, meaning that our opportunity is to inspire people that we work with and we're responsible to for the success of our communities and our organizations.

Bill: Thank you! I'm a big fan of servant leadership, so we have some alignment there.

Why did you choose healthcare as an occupation?

Mike: It's a very nice blend of the opportunity to help others, and the intellectual stimulus of the area of medicine which is constantly changing. There is so much that we don't know yet. I find that absolutely fascinating. Having something that, a discipline if you will, that we can continue to explore and grow and learn from and at the same time serve others that is very appealing to me.

Bill: Why did you specialize in infectious disease?

Mike: With infectious diseases you get to practice all specialties because it affects every other specialty within medicine. You have to know quite a bit about other specialties and how infections are potentially relevant in those areas. There is also the fact that it's an opportunity to immediately favorably impact people with certain infections that might not otherwise have improved.

Bill: Thank you for sharing that. You have had a variety of titles in your career, and your current role is as a consultant in antibiotic stewardship. You have also created an antibiotic stewardship program. Can you provide an overview of this antibiotic stewardship program?

Mike: Certainly. In Western South Dakota, for the last seventeen or eighteen years, we have had a program in place. The interesting aspect of this is, we're a rural frontier area. We have one microbiology lab in our referral hospital that serves a very large geographic area that is about 350 miles across. We can see how antibiotics and the changes in antibiotic use affect the bacteriology of our region. What we've been able to do is, based on that information, tell prescribers how to use antibiotics in a way that does not increase resistant bacteria. In fact, when there was the beginning of an increase we put changes in place that reversed that increase in resistant bacteria. For the last sixteen, seventeen years we've not had a rise in resistant bacteria in this region of the country.

Bill: Wow!

Mike: For that reason, we've thought that this model would be applicable to the other parts of the United States, if not all the United States to reverse the rise in resistant bacteria that most areas of the country have seen.

Bill: What is unique about this antibiotic stewardship program? It sounds like it applies to everyone, but what is unique about it for rural health?

Mike: What we've encountered is we work with many hospitals across the United States, in South Dakota and other states. When we interact with rural hospitals, particularly critical access hospitals. At a critical access hospital, there is the opportunity to influence the prescribing patterns of the whole community. About 70% of all antibiotics are used in the outpatient area. In rural areas, much of the hospital activities are tied into the community which provides the perfect opportunity to not only effect the inpatient prescribing of antibiotics, but the outpatient prescribing of antibiotics. This is key to protecting the safety of the community from resistant bacteria.

Bill: Interesting. One of the things that you and I talked about briefly a while back was the economics of antibiotic stewardship. Can you address that? What are the economics of antibiotic stewardship?

Mike: This is the one program that from a quality safety standpoint that can make things better or be safer for patients. When I was Chief Medical Officer, the question that always came up was, will this be better and safer for our patients. The next question that would follow is, how much is that going to cost us?

There always needs to be a cost benefit to pursue any program. In this particular case, you actually end up saving money by having an effective program in place because you can drive down total antibiotic use and also the amount of use for the more expensive antibiotics that have been developed. When we do that, we see a decrease in resistant bacteria, a decrease in readmissions and a decrease in a lot of the softer expenses that are harder to calculate. once a community calculates total antibiotic expenses, they often see pretty dramatic decreases in those costs. It's a quality safety program, and which also lowers costs, which, as a Chief Medical Officer, that is very appealing.

Bill: Sure, but in that process of driving down costs, part of the process increases costs because you have to do more diagnostic testing, don't you?

Mike: We do recommend increasing the emphasis on diagnostic testing because what we're finding is so many of the infections that people have, especially in the outpatient area, are viral infections. For instance, 90-95% of upper respiratory infections are viral, yet 75-80% of the time those patients are given antibiotics. There's a very significant opportunity to at least demonstrate by diagnostic testing that those infections are viral. This provides the opportunity to preserve the antibiotics for future times, when they may be specifically indicated for a bacterial infection.

Bill: Thank you.

There have been some recent scientific breakthroughs regarding our use of antibiotics. How does understanding these recent breakthroughs effect the use of antibiotics?

Mike: What is fascinating about medicine is there is so much yet to be learned. There's such complexity without understanding how the body works and how the body works in relationship to the environment. What we're beginning to understand is what's called the human microbiome. The National Institute of Health has stated that's the number two priority, after the human genome project, for ongoing research.

What the human microbiome is essentially is understanding that our body contains about forty trillion human cells. We also contain somewhere between forty and a hundred trillion bacterial cells. We have as much or more bacterial genetic material in our body than we do human genetic material. In the past, we had developed antibiotics in a strategic way nationally to treat all the possible causes of an infection. What that is called is a broad-spectrum antibiotic, meaning that not only is it going to treat the thing that we think is likely there but if we're wrong, it will cover some other things as well.

What we found is, that strategy has led to the development of resistant bacteria and worsening infectious complications like Clostridium difficile, also called C. diff. Because of that, we now know that a lot of our normal bacteria, probably about seven hundred to one, are helpful bacteria or what we call commensal bacteria, compared to one harmful or pathogenic bacteria.

We were damaging a lot of our protective bacteria that actually helps our immune system fight off the bad bacteria. By using the broad-spectrum antibiotics, it was a lot of friendly fire effect, if you will, in trying to treat the specific pathogen. That's another reason for improving our diagnostic test. If we can identify the specific pathogen, we can use an antibiotic specifically for that particular bacteria. That helps mitigate the risks of the infectious complications or resistant bacteria and helps preserve our antibiotics for future generations.

The data coming out of the human microbiome regarding our intestinal bacteria, our skin bacteria, and so forth, as far as all the other things that they may influence in our development and immunologic protection, it is fascinating to think that we are beginning to understand a lot of new science.

Bill: Yes, that is very interesting. I have always heard treating with a broadband spectrum of antibiotics referred to as shotgun medicine. Being a country boy and having blasted a few things with a shotgun, there is going to be collateral damage with that approach. It sounds like that metaphor still rings true to what you're talking about.

Mike: Absolutely.

Bill: What is the best strategy to conserve our precious resource of antibiotics, Dr. Keegan? For our children and our grandchildren, what do rural health leaders need to be doing differently in our strategy with antibiotics?

Mike: Initially, an awareness of what we're dealing with in clinical medicine is needed. When we're talking about hospital acquired infections, resistant bacteria, C. difficile, when we combine those and understand those are the things occurring in hospitals and nursing homes and occasionally in the outpatient area. If we look at the AIDS virus, tuberculosis and influenza, the three most common infections worldwide, hospital acquired infections with C. difficile are more common than all those combined.

What's happened is we've gotten bacteria to the point where there's some that we cannot even treat. The discussion centers are already entering the post-antibiotic era, meaning that we don't have antibiotics available to treat infections. If that were to occur we may not be able to treat with chemotherapy; we may not be able to do certain surgeries because the risk of infection growing to where we can't treat.

Rather than get there, what we advocate as a conservation program, meaning that in order to maintain our antibiotics for our children and our grandchildren. We need to use them very judiciously now. They are a very, very valuable resource for people that need them. But we've used them more as an insurance policy when we weren't sure whether the infection was a virus or a bacteria.

The approach is to, first of all, understand that, to be aware at the current state and what our risk is in the near term. Once we understand that and we commit to improving, then the measures are to reduce the use of broad spectrum antibiotics, to improve our diagnostic testing with rapid diagnostic testing so we can get the answers quickly and determine if we need to treat with an antibiotic. If we do, which specific antibiotic can we use that won't drive the harmful bacteria, the resistant bacteria?

The two biggest challenges in being successful are, first, how do you influence prescriber behavior? The way we found to be successful is to just share the evolving science. Physicians want to do what's best for their patients and having the latest state of the art strategies and information helps shore up their and their patients interest.

Second, patients come to expect antibiotics for any infection that occurs. How do you influence a patient by saying you have a viral infection because that sounds like it's a dismissive response to somebody that's feeling quite ill? The way to do that is to get a specific diagnosis. If we can diagnosis a specific virus and explain what that means, antibiotics are not beneficial for that. By not using them at this point when they don't help, we're preserving them to be effective in the future when you might need them.

Those two strategies respond to the two biggest challenges that we hear from almost every community we work in.

Bill: I know. I've gone to the doctor before, and it was determined that I had a viral infection, and the physician said well I can go ahead and give you an antibiotic if you want it just to be safe. You are saying that's not a good idea, correct?

Mike: Right. The second leading cause of trips to the emergency room is from medication misuse or medication complications. Second most common medications that are in that category are antibiotics. They're not nearly as safe as we would like to think.

Now that we know all these infectious complications such as Clostridium difficile or resistant bacteria associated. Then we're adding risks rather than any benefit, and so we have to make sure that we are providing more benefit than risks.

Bill: Thank you. The last time we talked, you mentioned a thirty-hospital collaborative that you're engaged with, with a focus on critical access hospitals. Can you share a bit about that?

Mike: Certainly, I'd be glad too. We just finished a year-long collaborative, and fifteen of the thirty hospitals are rural critical access hospitals. We found that to be a very nice compliment in that it gave us the opportunity to approach this challenge from a community wide perspective. In order words, if we are in a rural area we need to address what's going on in the long-term care facility, we need to address what's going on in the urgent care or the clinic, we may need to address what's going on at the developmental center, or the prison facility, or the school. We can work with the school nurse or the daycare center, whatever it might be where we can favorably influence the understanding and the responsibility of conserving antibiotic use.

The goal at the beginning was to decrease total antibiotic use and then broad spectrum antibiotic use, which are the main drivers of the resistant bacteria and the Clostridium difficile. At the end, we found that there was a 13-15% decrease of broad spectrum antibiotic use at the end of the year, whereas articles that have just come out, talking about how on whole, the US has not decreased antibiotics and has actually increased broad spectrum antibiotics. This was very remarkable because this was a state that came together and rather than just rationalizing the problem away said we want to do something about this, we want to create a safer environment for our communities and our citizens. It's just very, very impressive.

The other piece of that was that, of the thirty hospitals, only four didn't hit that broad-spectrum goal. If you just separate them out, the others actually decreased broad spectrum antibiotics in their facilities 25%, which is absolutely remarkable!

Bill: Wow, that seems rather significant.

Mike: It's very significant. I've not seen that done or reported anywhere else in the country. It's a wonderful achievement for that group of hospitals.

Bill: Well thank you for sharing that.

Dr. Keegan, what scares you most about the future of rural health? Would it be the use of antibiotics?

Mike: Actually, what scares me more is the underfunding of healthcare in the rural area.

I think often about how rural hospitals may be the number one employer in our smaller communities. As the number one employer, you hate to see the economic effect of being underfunded on the national or state level. I think there's a tremendous amount of value that our rural hospitals bring to their communities. I have witnessed it first-hand. I have truly enjoyed working with rural hospitals, and as I mentioned earlier, there's the opportunity to more directly affect the entire community.

Bill: What excites you the most about the future of rural health, Dr. Keegan?

Mike: Well, I think the people. The people that we've worked with are just wonderful. I think the number of hospitals, it may be the one hospital in particular, the board chair, one of the board members was the Mayor of the town, so when you're presenting to the hospital board you can directly connect with influencers in the community. At another, the Mayor was the Director of Marketing at the hospital. You can see how that just ties in nicely with everything that you're trying to accomplish at a rural hospital. It's the people caring about their neighbors. When there are improvements in healthcare, you can see it immediately translated into positive results. There's larger bureaucracy in larger areas, and we just don't tend to see that in rural areas where you can get things done quickly. That's a huge advantage with a challenge like this.

Bill: Thank you!

If people only take away one thing from this conversation, what should that be?

Mike: Our approach in the past has been, if we're not sure, let's use an antibiotic. The new approach needs to be, what proof is there that I have or need antibiotics because I know that there are risks and consequences. Rural health providers need to take advantage of newer diagnostic tests to confirm the diagnosis, to be not only responsible for your own care but understand how your decisions affect your neighbors and your family. In turn, making a good decision saves our antibiotics for our children and grandchildren.

Bill: Excellent! Thank you for sharing this important information, Dr. Keegan. You have some great experience and observations. Thank you for the great work you are doing in antibiotic stewardship.

Mike Huff

Mike Huff is CEO of Olney Hamilton Hospital. Mike is in charge of a hospital that has received national recognition for healthcare delivery. During our conversation, we discuss some of the things that make his hospital so successful. That includes the things needed to work with the staff to better understand what they need and where they're coming from, the work he did recruiting specialists for his community and the need for strategic planning. These, and many other helpful pieces of advice are found within this conversation with Mike Huff.

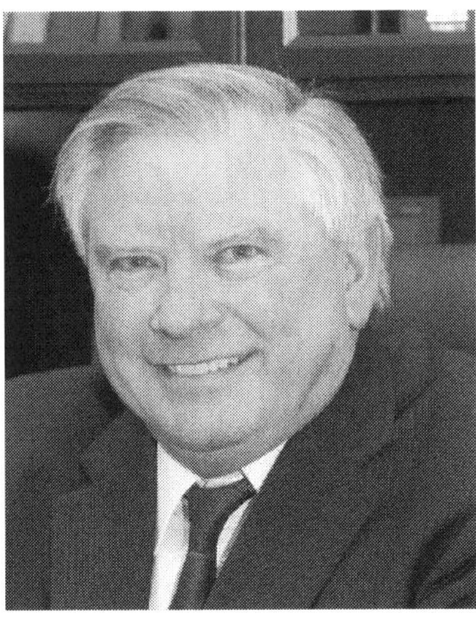

Bill: Mike Huff is the CEO of Olney Hamilton Hospital. Olney Hamilton Hospital is a critical access hospital located in Olney, Texas, which is in the north central part of Texas, about halfway between Dallas and Amarillo. Mike has been the CEO of Olney Hamilton Hospital since 2011. Prior to that, he was the president of the east Georgia division of St. Joseph's health system in Atlanta, Georgia, and president and CEO of St. Joseph's at East Georgia, a critical access hospital.

Under his leadership at Olney Hamilton Hospital, the hospital has been recognized as one of the best places to work by Modern Healthcare. They've also been recognized for overall excellence in outcomes by the National Organization of State Offices of Rural Health, and iVantage Health Analytics. Just recently, Olney Hamilton Hospital was recognized as a 'Top 20 Critical Access Hospital' by the National Rural Health Association. They provide that recognition based on nine indices: inpatient market share, outpatient market share, population risk, cost, charge, quality, outcomes, patient perspectives, and financial stability. Mike, please correct me if I'm wrong, but I think this is the second year in a row that your hospital has been recognized as a 'Top 20 Critical Access Hospital', is that correct?

Mike: That is correct, Bill, and thank you so much for the opportunity to talk about our great little hospital here. Last year we were honored to be recognized as one of the top 100 rural hospitals in the nation. Then again, this year, we got the very distinguished honor of being one of the top critical access hospitals in the area of quality. We are very excited about these awards and recognition.

Bill: Looking at all of the information that I could've shared about you and your hospital, the list is so long that I had to sort out what to include and not to include. You've had a very distinguished career in healthcare, and you've done an incredible job at Olney Hamilton Hospital in the last few years.

There're a lot of career paths that you could've chosen, Mike. Why did you choose healthcare as an occupation?

Mike: Very good question. Actually, I've been asked that many times. As we were growing up, my mom was a nurse, and I recall, back in the day, we would go up to the hospital, take her to work, or go see her. I always looked at hospitals as a place where you not only went when you needed healthcare, but it was a place of employment. It was intriguing, and I never lost sight of that. Over time, as I was finishing my education, I evolved to that, and it's a very fulfilling career path. I've never looked back. Every day is a new day, and I get excited getting up in the morning and going to work. I have been very blessed with this particular career path.

Bill: That's wonderful. Why rural health specifically?

Mike: I've been in all size hospitals, major hospitals, midsize hospitals. I had my first taste of rural health when I was in Georgia. There's just something about working in a smaller hospital, the family-like atmosphere of the hospital and the employees. Everyone reaches out to help each other and stay focused on the patients and quality patient care. It has probably been the most rewarding times in my life. I know without a doubt, since I've been here, I've never had more fun in my

25+ years in this business than I have working in a rural hospital. It is one of the best decisions that I've made.

Bill: When you get out of bed every day energized and going to work is fun, it's no wonder that your hospital has been recognized so much since you've taken over the role of CEO.

What is your definition of leadership?

Mike: Leadership really can be defined as how well you can work with your team, and I mean work with them. You don't lead the team, you work with them and mentor them to achieve your goals. Not only to achieve the goals, but to help them achieve in the manner that you're setting the pace. I always like to explain to my staff, "yes, we want really good patient care, but we also should swing for the fence every once in a while. Let's see if we can do something better than anyone else. Let's set the standard where everyone else will call us and say 'what in the world are you guys doing out there? That's great'". They love that. They like the idea. Let's pick something to be the best at it. When you have your team all focused on that goal, I'll tell you again, it gets back to having fun at what you're doing. It's really exciting to work in that environment.

Bill: Mentoring is so important. When you are mentored or you're mentoring others
, it has such a powerful impact on so many aspects of life. The Major League Baseball Wild Card playoffs are going on right now as we having this conversation, so I like the analogy of swinging for the fence. As one of my friends said, "be careful, if you set the bar too low, you just might achieve it". Setting the bar high is a great thing.

You've had some great success as a leader. What would you say your top leadership strength is?

Mike: Probably my ability to relate to the staff and understand the staff so they can, in turn, feel like they can trust management and know that, if they have issues, we work together as a family. You're only as good as the people you have around you. If you work diligently towards that and provide a clear articulation of what our goals and our standards are, people know that going into it. A career in healthcare doesn't fit everybody. Healthcare is a unique business.

I've always said that anybody who works in healthcare has a special place in their heart, because if you're in it just for the money or whatever else, those people get weeded out pretty fast. The people who get into healthcare and stay there, it's because they like helping others. That's a fundamental piece of their being. Their completeness, if you will, is the fact that they can go home at the end of the day and say, "I really helped somebody today". When you get a group of people like that who set their sights on high quality goals and patient outcomes, that's really exciting to watch.

Bill: Did you grow up in a rural community?

Mike: I grew up in a medium sized community. But one of the biggest impressions of my life was in a rural area. My grandfather was a farmer and rancher. When my folks would go on vacation, I would always ask, "well just take me to my granddads and leave me there". I got to love the rural area and what it means and their values. That's something that's always been very important to me and has been a driver for me. My grandfather used to say "one of the best compliments in life is when you do something for someone, you don't tell them, and they find out about it maybe years later. You do it because it's the right thing to do". I've always felt like people in healthcare have that same philosophy if you will. That same 'let's work together to help people' philosophy.

Bill: That's great! The reason I asked you that is because, some people who did grow up in a more urban area, instead of a rural area, do incredibly great things while others struggle. It sounds like you made that transition early in life with your grandpa.

Mike: You make a good point there, Bill. Rural does have its limitations, and it certainly has its frustrations and challenges. I think to be successful and to make sure your employees are successful, you just have to recognize that. Again, you pick those areas that you can do, but you do them very well. You don't try to be everything to everyone. What you can do, you just focus on that, look at best practices and set your standards.

Bill: We've mentioned some of the awards that your hospital has been recognized for, including the 'Top 20 Critical Access Hospital for Quality' just last month. When you arrived back in 2011, what was the state of affairs at the hospital?

Mike: I would say the hospital was going through some transition. There had been some change in some of the key positions at the hospital. There were some questions about who reported to who and why they reported to them and 'do I really have to do this'. I think there was a leadership void at that time. It was a good hospital and it was a good staff. I think we essentially have probably the majority of the same staff. I worked very hard at putting together a really good senior management team. You want to put a team together that, if you're not in or you're not available, the wheels don't fall off. Other people can just pick it up and run with it, and you never miss a lick. Like I said, you're only as good as the people you have around you.

Bill: The management team that you put together, with the change of leadership and the transition you were talking about, there had to be some cultural change involved in that. How did you change the culture?

Mike: Absolutely, there was cultural change. There was quite a bit of change. It was just setting the standards and staying true to what you believe in. People are hesitant to change, especially in a smaller hospital. Change can be such a huge factor in someone's life. I've been doing it this way for ten years. Let's try something different. I don't know if it'll work. We won't know until we try. You hold their hands, take baby steps, you stay with your plan. You stay with your goals and targets.

Most people will eventually come along if they know they're being treated fairly, and they also know that you're asking their input. If they say "well, this won't work", well tell me why. What can we do to make it work? What're your ideas? I always tell my department managers, "no one knows your job better than you. If we're doing something you feel is inhibiting you from giving good patient care, tell me what we need to change. What do we do differently? Show me how it works best for you." If they feel a part of it, and they feel like they can effectuate their own changes, they buy into it more readily, and it does go a little smoother.

Bill: Those are some powerful questions to ask, and those questions only matter when you listen to what the answers are.

Mike: Absolutely.

Bill: Your hospital has received a lot of recognition. You talked about change in the culture. You talked about the leadership change. What else have you done that has led to your hospital being so successful?

Mike: We've worked very diligently with our medical staff. When I got here, they were in a pretty rundown clinic and weren't close to the hospital. We built them a brand-new clinic right across the street from the hospital. They love that, but our patients in our community really have enjoyed that. It's been a good financial move. We've occupied that since 2012, and we've seen between three and five percent growth year over year since we've occupied that new clinic. We put in a wellness center, again to show the community, "we're reaching out to you. We're going to offer these types of services that will help you and the rest of the community." That has really made a major impact with that.

The board, just like the employees and medical staff, requires continuing education. The board's been here a long time. They love this hospital. They are very engaged. It took some education with the board, and saying "here's some things we can do that will improve patient care and improve outcomes and improve employee satisfaction," and they were quite receptive. They bought into some of this, gave it a shot, and said "okay, let's try it." When you have a board willing to buy into your ideas and work with you, that is everything, to have a supportive board.

Bill: It makes a huge difference, doesn't it?

Mike: It does.

Bill: Well thank you, Mike! So far, you have shared some great information.

Bill: Is there anything else that's unique that you have done as a rural health leader that worked out?

Mike: When we looked at what services the hospital currently provides and what services are we sending out of the community, we found several areas that would fit our community and our hospital that we could do a very good job of. It would help the hospital financially, but it would also keep our community and our patients from having to drive an hour, and sometimes two hours, to get that care. We have developed many programs like cardiopulmonary rehab, for example, and enhanced our rehab department where we now have a full complement of not just physical therapy, but we also have speech therapy and occupational therapy.

For a rural area, that is really something. It's difficult to find those type of therapies in rural areas. We've seen significant growth in those services. I have recruited specialists from some of the major communities who make rotating visits here. We have cardiology now, we have orthopedics, oncology and gastroenterology. Those specialists come through, and that's really been a godsend for some of our elder community members who find it very difficult to have to travel to seek those types of specialists.

Bill: Absolutely! I don't know about you, but I like to talk about the stuff I tried that didn't work. Sometimes, we try new things that don't always work out the way that we planned, and sometimes those are even more powerful lessons to learn from. Is there anything that you tried that didn't necessarily work out the way that you had hoped?

Mike: A bunch. Getting back to our sports analogy, Babe Ruth was the top home-run hitter, but what most people don't say is he also had more strikeouts than anyone else.

Bill: Exactly.

Mike: Sure, you get up to the plate and strike out sometimes. I remember at one hospital, we had started a hospitalist program, and we started it around one of the internal medicine physicians that had grown up in the community. She was an excellent, well liked physician. It was a huge success, partially because everyone knew her. She was a good doctor. Then, she got an opportunity, and unfortunately, we lost her. She went on to continue her education. I just said, "well, I'll just replace her". It was a failure. No one wanted to use them anymore. It's not that the doctor that I brought in wasn't good, it was just that no one knew him. It gets back to you're only as good as the people you have around you. Ultimately, I had to discontinue that program because it wasn't working out. That was a real lesson learned. It's all about having the right people.

Bill: Interesting lesson. What do you think that rural health leaders need to do differently?

Mike: They have to be flexible. I hate to beat this analogy to death, but some of things that Yogi Bear used to say, "when you come to the fork in the road, take it". That's kind of the way I feel now in this environment with all of the changes and everything uncertain. You have to be able to adapt. The only certain thing in this business is what I'm going to see today is going to be different from what I see tomorrow.

You've got to figure out and marshal the resources that you have. We have great state associations here. We have a rural association of hospitals called TORCH. We have Texas Hospital Association, and there are other national associations. Use all of the resources you have, and reach out and ask people "how are you doing this?" Try to manage on a day to day basis.

Another thing that always works well, you've got to have at least a three, if not a five-year strategic plan. I certainly wouldn't go over five. I think three would probably be outdated these days. You have to have a road map, recognizing that will probably change by the time the print is dry. Have a road map, know where you're going, and then just modify it as you need it to get there. Those type of things I would say.

Bill: Yes, and you were also supposed to say "listen to *Rural Health Leadership Radio™"* too.

Mike: That's right, that's one of those resources. Definitely, because you do reach out and find people who have had successes in an area and best practices. You're absolutely, right.

Bill: What scares you the most about the future of rural health?

Mike: The shift in demographics both at the state and national level. It hasn't been that long ago that rural had a great deal of clout in Congress. Most of the demographic change is people in rural moving to the urbans. Your political clout now resides in urban areas. To an extent, the rurals don't have a voice at the state level or the national level. You're pretty well subject to the whims of those that do have a voice. It makes it interesting.

Bill: There is a lot of concern about all the rural hospitals that are at the risk of closing. That's a very legitimate concern, 'do we have a voice at the capital or the state capitals?'

There is also a lot of excitement about the future. What excites you the most about the future of rural health?

Mike: There will always be a need for rural health, especially in states like Texas. It's very wide, and you may travel two hours and not see anything but straps in the road and fence post.

Bill: I've been on some of those drives. I know what you mean.

Mike: There will always be a need for rural health. The exciting part is to make sure that you will be there for the next ten years, 20 years, and 30 years. You may not look like you do today, but you will be there and still providing the essence of your mission, and that is the best healthcare that you can provide to your community.

Bill: Very important. You've been doing this for a while now, you've had some great success in your career at both larger hospitals, and then in the last ten years in rural health. Are you having fun? Are you looking to retire?

Mike: I really can't see myself retiring right now. Yes, I'm having fun, I'm having a blast. Obviously, there're some days more frustrating than others, but overall, like I said I still enjoy getting up and going to work in the morning. The retirement piece of it, if I get to a point where number one, I'm not having fun or number two, I'm not able to make positive changes, then I guess I could look at either doing something else or perhaps retirement. Right now, things are working. I'm having fun. Retirement is not in the near future.

Bill: Good! I think a lot of people in the Olney, Texas, are happy to hear that.

One question I meant to ask you earlier is about advocacy. What role should a rural hospital CEO have in advocacy?

Mike: I think this would fit any hospital CEO. With all of the changes in healthcare, and the fact that so much of the federal deficit and the spending at the federal level is related to healthcare in some aspect. If you're not involved, and you're not actively involved in your local, state and federal political arena and plugged into advocacy, then it's like if you don't vote, you don't have a right to complain. I think now, more than I've ever seen in my career, that's one of the most important aspects of this.

I know it feels like 'well I don't think I can make a difference'. Whether you feel that way or not, if you're making your concerns known, if you're plugged in and you're talking to your state rep or your national rep, at least you're educated on the subject. You've educated yourself, and you know the issues. That's half the battle, just knowing the information and knowing where the goal posts are. I think that's probably one of the most important things I would tell a young person wanting to enter this business right now. You're going to have to learn how to be a politician whether you like it or not, just for survival.

Bill: That's interesting. That leads me to my last question. What advice would you have for a CEO just starting out in rural healthcare?

Mike: Basically, I look back on the way I did it. If you have a burning drive in your gut, and this is something you're excited about, follow your dreams. There will always be a need for talented healthcare professionals. Don't be afraid to change. Don't be afraid of failure. Learn from your mistakes. Pick yourself up, dust your pants off, and keep going until you figure out a way to make it work. Never underestimate the power of your employees, those type of things. Set yourself goals and stick to your guns. It's going to be tough, but it's a very rewarding career, and you'll never look back.

Bill: Mike, that sounds like some great advice. I want to thank you for sharing your thoughts, observations and experiences in rural health.

Terry Hill

Terry Hill is the Executive Director of Rural Health Innovations, located in Duluth, Minnesota. Terry covers several issues during our conversation, including a hospital reopening a movie theater to cut down on car accidents. The primary focus of our conversation is with regard to the shift to delivering value in healthcare. Instead of focusing on volume, healthcare facilities are now focusing on the value of the care. Terry provides a look at how this change is happening and the effects it will have.

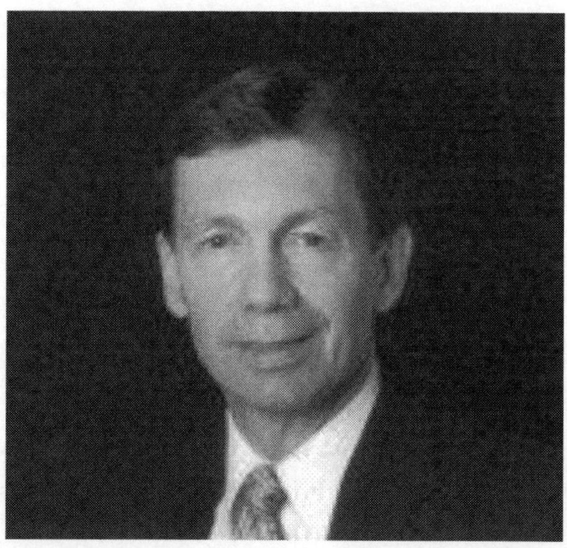

Bill: Terry Hill is the Executive Director of Rural Health Innovations. Terry is also the founder and Senior Advisor of the National Rural Health Resource Center. Terry's role as the Senior Advisor at the Rural Health Resource Center is focused on rural health leadership and policy. Terry has more than 30 years of experience in rural healthcare, working with rural health leaders in 47 states. He's facilitated seven National Summit Meetings, written dozens of published articles, led 11 national demonstration projects in rural health, and helped develop three national healthcare delivery models, critical access hospitals, frontier extended stay clinics, and frontier community health integration models.

Terry has been teaching management and leadership in the MBA program for rural health leadership at The College of St. Scholastica for 11 years. He also teaches a course in American Health Policy at the University of Minnesota Medical School. Last year, Terry received the President's Award from the National Rural Health Association. Terry is a true expert on rural health leadership, and I'm very honored to talk with him. Welcome, Terry.

Terry: Thank you very much, Bill.

Bill: Terry, I know that you and I, when we've talked in the past, we've talked a lot about leadership, so let me ask you, what's your definition of leadership?

Terry: For me, leadership is really the process of serving others. I've always looked at our organization's major purpose which is to serve rural communities, for example, and as a leader of this organization, I've seen my primary role of serving the staff and serving our organizations so it in turn can serve others. As I think I've told you in the past, I'm a huge fan of and try to practice servant leadership, and I believe it's the most effective leadership style that I've seen.

Bill: Yes. We are both kindred spirits when it comes to the idea of servant leadership, so thank you for sharing your definition. Terry, why did you choose healthcare as an occupation?

Terry: I chose it, Bill, largely because it was an opportunity to provide service. For a while, I provided service directly to clients and patients, but there seemed to be an opportunity to work upstream a bit and perhaps make an impact on healthcare policy. I thought that perhaps we could make a wider contribution. I enjoy the patient care and the customer service, the direct provision of that service, but it became an opportunity to do something in healthcare, it's been a privilege to be a part of serving others. I think healthcare, teaching and a few other occupations really have an opportunity to make a huge impact. I think I recognized that and I wanted to be a part of that.

Bill: Why rural health?

Terry: First of all, I grew up in a very tiny town of about 80 people in the middle of Alaska so I come from that sort of background. I grew up with a native population in Alaska and for me, it's always been about the country and being out in the woods. The other thing about rural is it's just the historic underdog. It's in the minority. We have more problems and issues there. And finally, I really like the spirit and the innovation of the people that I work with that are very often up against challenges that our city counterparts don't have.

Bill: Yes. It's a unique aspect of healthcare, dealing with rural health. Why do you think that leadership is so important in rural health?

Terry: We've done research, and I've participated in quite a bit of research, particularly with the University of Minnesota and here at the Center as well. It's become very clear over the course of my career that leadership is the single most important determinant of success for virtually any endeavor for any organization. It's always the most critical variable so, for example, when we studied rural health networks, we came to the conclusion that those networks that had great leaders virtually always had very good, if not great results. Where leadership struggled, we found it was very rare to see the organization overcome struggling leadership and produce excellent results. The sustainability of excellent leadership is crucial to sustainable outcomes.

I could point, for example, to the Baldridge framework that we use here at the Center where leadership is basically valued more than any other determinant of the eventual outcomes. In fact, the leadership component has doubled the worth of any other single component, they have six all together, leading to extraordinary outcomes. Of those six components, leadership has double the amount of points in regard to the Baldridge Quality Award. It's so clear to me how important leadership is.

Bill: You've seen that firsthand?

Terry: Absolutely. It's inspiring. You can step into a hospital, for example, and within the first 5 to 10 minutes, you can get a pretty good feel for the type of leadership that is there. You can tell this partially from the degree of customer service, to the degree to which the staff is happy and customer-focused. That is all a product of leadership.

Bill: Interesting observations. Since leadership is so important, what is the most important leadership strength that rural health leaders need?

Terry: I think there are a couple. I didn't come up with just one. One of them would have to be perseverance. Perseverance means, in essence, you're going to go through the good times and the bad times and you've got to be able to be tough and persevere through those. If you are the leader of the organization, folks are going to look to you when things go wrong. You have to set the example of being strong and being optimistic. I always look at resilience as a very important factor. I'd also put the whole concept of humility, not needing to take credit for the successes, trying to really focus in on the "we" rather than the "I." Humility is important too. In essence, the leader naturally gets a whole lot of the credit for the work done by the staff, and I think deflecting their credit to the degree possible is always a good idea.

Bill: You're listing the top two leadership strengths that rural leaders need to have is perseverance and/or resilience along with humility. Great! Thank you for zeroing in on those.

What about the importance of delivering value? Healthcare is all about value and shifting to being all about value anyway. What about the importance of delivering value?

Terry: I think it's terrific news that we're moving in that direction. If you think about it, healthcare has been thrown into the business arena and for quite some time, we were rewarding volume rather than value. In a payment system that's based in value, we are basically going to reward quality, customer service and cost becomes a factor as well. Two of the most important issues right now with the American healthcare system are the extremely high costs, far higher than any other country in the world, and then the whole issue of quality and not being able to have anywhere close to the kind of quality outcomes and patient safety outcomes we need. As we shift the system to value, we're now rewarding for high quality and reasonable cost. That system change itself is going to have a profound impact, not just on the delivery system, but on the experience of patients and their families.

Bill: Do you think that most rural health leaders are prepared for this shift to deliver value?

Terry: I think rural health leaders have always had to be fairly resilient. I try to get across as I talk to rural health leaders that this profound change is going to be challenging to both rural and urban leaders, but generally, one of the real strengths of a rural leader is that they're generally overseeing much smaller organizations that can be more mobile. They can change more quickly. I'm not sure that rural leaders are fully prepared, but I think just in terms of the kind of ingenuity that they've needed, the very challenges they've faced already, they are in a good position to be successful in this new environment. To be really clear about my opinion on that, I think rural health is going to make out very well in this new value payment delivery system, particularly if we move and take advantage of the time that is there to prepare and move forward.

Bill: Thank you. Another hot topic these days is population management. Can you share your thoughts on population management as it applies to rural health?

Terry: In the past, the responsibility of population health management was given to public health, which is woefully underfunded and under-resourced. Public health made huge contributions to water quality, immunization and disease prevention, but it never had the resources to truly make a profound impact on the overall health of the public. What I see now is public health has all of these new allies with hospitals and clinics. Healthcare providers, in general, are being incentivized to keep people healthy to begin with and then to manage chronic illnesses like diabetes, before it becomes severe, before it requires hospitalization, before it requires amputation. Population health is going to benefit from the innovations within the entire healthcare industry. We are working with healthcare providers willing to partner with their communities, with the patients and the public at large to produce better outcomes. I'm optimistic that since the financing is now supporting these initiatives, it's actually going to happen.

Bill: Thank you, Terry. It's important as our healthcare system continues to evolve to try new things, and in that light, can you talk about something unique that either you've done or you've witnessed another rural health leader do that they implemented that worked?

Terry: I remember a hospital administrator in a Northern Minnesota hospital who really tried to make an impact on community wellbeing. This happened way before hospitals got paid for population health or got paid for the kind of services that I think we're going to find support for financially in the future. This particular community had recently closed down its movie theater. The movie theater was a source of entertainment for this small town. Teenagers and young people started driving to International Falls, far north of their community, to see movies. Because these movies were held late at night, these kids were driving late at night. They were experiencing a number of accidents and several kids had died as a result. The hospital administrator looked at the responsibilities of the hospital and thought, "We could be doing more."

The hospital, which had some cash reserves, was able to buy the old movie theater and start funding it, subsidizing it, so the young people in the town could stay locally to watch a movie. To my knowledge, that hospital is still operating that movie theater. I see that as an outstanding example of a hospital and a leader taking on responsibilities over and above what has historically been the role of hospitals. This is not an isolated incident.

I could tell you at least another dozen stories about hospitals that have really reached out and dealt with social issues, dealt with public health issues, have started programs. I know quite a number right now that are doing a really extraordinary job dealing with opioid addiction. That's just one example. It always comes to mind because I was so impressed with that CEO's leadership. The contribution to the community was fewer accidents, fewer young people dying. It's just one little example, but it always impressed me.

Bill: That is a great story. How many hospitals do you know that are investing in movie theaters?

Can you talk about something that you've seen a rural health leader try that didn't work out the way they had planned?

Terry: I think what has happened so often in the past is that leaders with the kind of motivation that I talked about to do something in the community really reached out and put a significant amount of hospital resources into programs designed to support the general community or the population itself. Part of the issue though is that when that sort of expenditure takes places and then when we see difficult financial times, like cutbacks in federal funding, Medicaid funding, or private insurance funding, it's difficult for hospitals or healthcare organizations to sustain those sorts of community contributions. Hospice and nursing homes that have historically been there were discontinued due to those cutbacks. I have frequently seen hospitals make a good faith effort to make contributions, but because there was no funding available for it, no source of revenue for it, have to cut back in that regard.

That's changing, and now what we're seeing is keeping the population healthy. Value based reimbursement provides incentive and financial support for the very first time to do the socially responsible or the right thing. I'm very enthusiastic about that. We have enabled great contributions from our rural healthcare providers and we are also starting to identify a source of revenue to support those.

Bill: Thank you for sharing that. When you were talking about the unique things that you've seen rural health leaders do that worked out well, you gave us a great story about the movie theater. When we were talking about that, you mentioned that you've seen some unique things done regarding opioid use. That is a really big problem these days. Can you expand on that?

Terry: What we're seeing, especially in some areas of the country, opioid addiction is rampant. And of course, opioid addiction frequently leads to heroin addiction. It's a problem that has at least some of its base in the pain medication system that has been in this country for years and years. In essence, the prescribing of opioids for pain relief has been a double-edged sword. On the one hand, it's provided great relief to folks that have been in pain. On the other side of that, it's often led to very dangerous addictions and what seems to be increasing problems in our high schools with our young people in particular.

One of the other things that comes out of these new value models is that for the first time, providers really get a more comprehensive look at the complete medical experience of their patients. In the past, it has not been possible because there has been an incomplete story that the medical providers have. They have been unable to tell if somebody gets pain medication from their clinic and then goes to another clinic. They can do this sort of shopping around for pain medication and get multiple prescriptions. I've seen one patient who was able to get 13 separate sources for pain medication. I believe that they probably didn't use it all themselves. They were basically selling part of it as well. It's a very, very serious problem. It now exceeds motor vehicle accidents as a source of death for people under 30. The solution is going to require a multifaceted, more community-based approach and is going to require that hospitals and clinics work together with police, perhaps churches and mental health agencies.

Bill: Thank you for diving into that. What do you think that rural health leaders need to be doing differently?

Terry: We're in a really precarious position right now because of the diversity of our funding. What we note is that our critical access hospitals are still getting cost-based reimbursement, but many of them are now participating in value-based models which give a different source of funding. What I think is imperative at the moment is that all rural healthcare organizations begin to prepare for value based reimbursement. It doesn't mean that we're going to abandon or not really strive for keeping cost based reimbursement for critical access hospitals, or some of the advantages we have in rural health clinics, or community health centers, but we've got to develop the skills for care coordination. We have got to be thinking about how we're going to manage patient information bases. We've got to prepare the staff. We have to be working as more coordinated teams. We need to be looking across service delivery systems, not just at the hospital or clinic, but the handoff of patients from one service sector to the other.

It is taking a balanced approach, preparing for the future without getting too far ahead of ourselves in terms of preparation, and then making a planned transition from one payment system to the other. It is going to vary state by state, I think. It may very well vary from one hospital to the next or from one clinic to the next, but it is absolutely the time to be thinking about and incorporating into our strategic planning all of these concepts of value and population health management.

Bill: Thank you for sharing that information about what we need to do differently.

What excites you the most about the future of rural health, Terry?

Terry: What really excites me is the fact that after a lot of butting our heads against the wall, we are redesigning our healthcare system and paying finally for the right things and that is value. I'm excited that I see a lot of great innovation out there and terrific leadership. I see a future role for rural hospitals, a super significant role for rural clinics, and I believe that another real exciting aspect of that is the new payment models will want to keep the patients and the care delivery as local as possible.

Bill: Thank you, Terry. We've talked a lot about a lot of different topics, delivering value, population health, hospital investing into a movie theater, etc. If there's only one thing people take away from our conversation, what should that one thing be?

Terry: I would say that rural health has a very significant role and a real opportunity to help change the American healthcare system. We have an opportunity to be innovative. We have an opportunity to provide even greater services to our community. The time is now to prepare for that transition. Leadership is going to be the single most important determinant of what will be either a successful transition into value and population health or an unsuccessful transition.

Bill: Terry Hill, thank you so much for having this conversation, sharing your thoughts and your observations and expertise in rural health.

Bill Auxier

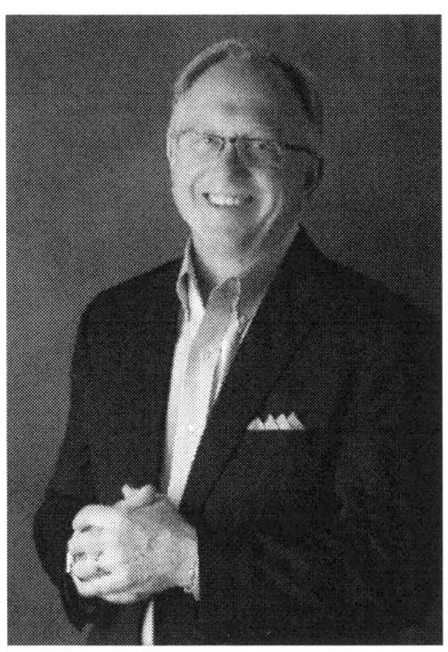

Bill Auxier, Ph.D., is the creator and host of the podcast *Rural Health Leadership Radio™.* He is a contributing author to the *Wall Street Journal* Best-seller *Masters of Success*, author of the award-winning best-seller *To Lead, Follow*, a speaker, founder of the Dynamic Leadership Academy™ for Rural Health, Adjunct Assistant Professor at the University of Maryland University College and 35-year veteran of the healthcare industry. Bill assists rural healthcare leaders achieve greatness through leadership development consulting and coaching. He does this by utilizing what he has learned about leadership in the real world combined with what he has learned about leadership in the academic world. In the real world, Bill started his career in healthcare as a nurse's aide in a small rural hospital. From there, he worked his way up to become the CEO of a medical device manufacturer with global distribution.

Bill and his wife, Elise, have two grown children, a rescue dog named Pepper, and reside in Tampa, FL.

Made in the USA
Columbia, SC
16 June 2018